MW00343520

Spatial Epidemiological Approaches in Disease Mapping and Analysis

Spatial Epidemiological Approaches in Disease Mapping and Analysis

Poh-Chin Lai
Fun-Mun So
Ka-Wing Chan

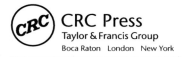

CRC Press
Taylor & Francis Group
Boca Raton   London   New York

CRC Press is an imprint of the
Taylor & Francis Group, an **informa** business

CRC Press
Taylor & Francis Group
6000 Broken Sound Parkway NW, Suite 300
Boca Raton, FL 33487-2742

© 2009 by Taylor & Francis Group, LLC
CRC Press is an imprint of Taylor & Francis Group, an Informa business

International Standard Book Number-13: 978-1-4200-4546-8 (Hardcover)

Library of Congress Cataloging-in-Publication Data

Lai, Poh C.
    Spatial epidemiological approaches in disease mapping and analysis / Poh Chin Lai, Fun Mun So, Ka Wing Chan.
        p. ; cm.
    Includes bibliographical references and index.
    ISBN 978-1-4200-4546-8 (hardback : alk. paper)
    1. Medical geography. 2. Medical mapping. 3. Geographic information systems. I. So, Fun Mun. II. Chan, Ka Wing. III. Title.
    [DNLM: 1. Epidemiologic Methods. 2. Geographic Information Systems. 3. Geography. WA 950 L185s 2009]

RA792.L35 2009
614.4'2--dc22   2008025463

Visit the Taylor & Francis Web site at
http://www.taylorandfrancis.com

and the CRC Press Web site at
http://www.crcpress.com

Contents

Foreword

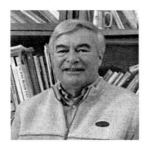

This handbook of spatial epidemiological approaches in disease mapping and analysis fills a gap in the book literature that remains rather glaringly open after the publication, fairly recently, of three books on spatial epidemiology[1-3] — all written by epidemiologists and spatial statisticians. This gap covers the characteristics of geospatial information and methods and the procedures that are typically followed to implement applications in public health in real situations. Most applications of GIS in the literature are described as projects related to data unique to their project. It is easy to see how people with an interest in public health problems in their geographic context will come away from this literature with the mistaken impression that every case they work with must be developed as if it were such a project. *Spatial Epidemiological Approaches in Disease Mapping and Analysis* shows the future path for people who work on public health problems in a particular country or region to be the construction of a geospatial data framework for that region — usually in cooperation with other users of geospatial data in their region — and then for each problem as it arises, to examine the most appropriate geospatial scale with which to pursue their questions of interest. In case such a common-sense approach should appear unexceptional, readers of the three books referenced will note that their point of departure generally begins with the geospatial data prespecified and the task at hand to be selection of methods to match the data at hand. This handbook turns this last approach on its head. It starts with the premise that every public health question that has a geographic dimension needs to be evaluated first in terms of the levels of spatial resolution needed for its examination. It notes how the availability of data often constrains the ability for ideal spatial resolution levels to be pursued but, nevertheless, leads the user down the logical decision-making path of examining the geography first before pursuing the spatial–statistical relationships of interest. With this approach, the geospatial horse leads the spatial epidemiological cart; as well should!

The book begins with the establishment of the concept of a geospatial data system and discusses how such a system is built from often quite separate, disparate sources. It then makes the critical distinction between point- and area-based spatial data systems and discusses the kinds of methods of mapping and spatial data analysis associated with each system. Problems of spatial misalignment of zonal data and consequences of the different shapes and sizes of spatial data units are discussed. A notable feature of the book is the template followed, which consists of brief descriptions of analysis methods, key references to literature that discusses the methods, and illustrations of applications of the methods to real data sets in Hong Kong or Thailand. Software available in the public domain is used in these illustrations in most cases. The final chapter concludes with a wide-ranging overview of many applications of GIS to contemporary health problems. This handbook sets the stage for a future handbook that no doubt will address the operational procedures needed to implement dynamic, real-time, rapid response, GIS-based health surveillance systems.

This handbook is a very timely and useful contribution to much-needed instructional resources in spatial epidemiology. It is a welcome addition and will find a global audience as befits the global challenge of improving the abilities of health departments to address public health problems in their geographic context.

Gerard Rushton
University of Iowa
Iowa City, Iowa

References

1. Elliott, P., Wakefield, J.C., Best, N.G., and Briggs, D.J. Eds., *Spatial Epidemiology: Methods and Applications*, Oxford University Press, Oxford, 2000.
2. Schabenberger, O., and Gotway, C.A., Statistical Methods for Spatial Data Analysis, Chapman & Hall, CRC Press, Boca Raton, FL, 2005.
3. Waller, L.A., and Gotway, C.A., *Applied Spatial Statistics for Public Health Data*, Wiley, Hoboken, NJ, 2004.

Foreword

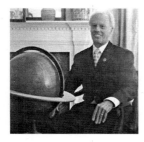

As we begin the twenty-first century, the field of geography has taken on heightened importance through many new developments in computer-based digital technologies. None of these could be more significant than the use of GIS to advance the role of location- or place-based science. For students and practitioners alike, especially those working on earth, social, behavioral, and biomedical sciences, the demand for bringing the GIS toolkit to bear beneficially upon these many disciplines has grown exponentially and worldwide. Thus, the timing is excellent for this handbook, which provides a well-balanced mix of instructional and operational procedures to help bridge, through a GIS environment, geographic science and epidemiology.

Spatial Epidemiological Approaches in Disease Mapping and Analysis reflects a dedicated effort by a team of Hong Kong University geographers to help satisfy the demand for applied approaches to solve contemporary spatial epidemiological research challenges. What makes the handbook an exciting accomplishment is that this body of work has applicability on any disease or public heath condition, whether taking place on a global, national, community, or parcel scale. It provides a framework for using epidemiological data that have been spatially empowered with geographic identifiers. The end result is a handbook, based on geographic science, that will aid researchers in the mapping and analysis of epidemiological and public health information using GIS.

The foundation for using GIS in spatial epidemiology is established in the beginning chapters as the reader is introduced to GIS, its concepts and operations, and basic GIS data models and how these relate to epidemiological data having geographic properties. Here the reader is instructed as to the components and functionalities of GIS and approaches for GIS organization and operation. Common data models for spatial analysis and key concepts of data attributes, geocoding, topology, and data aggregation are examined.

The reader then is prepared for the integration of geocoded health information (e.g., asthma hospitalizations from both Thailand and Hong Kong, severe acute respiratory syndrome cases from Hong Kong, dengue from Thailand) into the GIS and the ensuing spatial analytic and presentation methods used by geographers. Navigating the intersection of geography with epidemiological observation, including contributions from the disciplines of statistics, cartography (map design and visualization), and psychology (human cognition), reflects the complexity behind disease mapping and analysis and becomes the mainstay and key contribution of the book. Here the reader is guided in the use of geospatial analytic freeware (download-able from the Internet) with which disease occurrence data can be examined for spatial randomness, dependencies, pattern, and trend.

A welcome inclusion to the handbook is the instructional clarity in the treat-ment of spatial–statistical techniques. Here spatial epidemiological data are subjected to statistical rigor and advanced methodological testing, which help to remove the analytic constraints of spatial masks or boundaries. Conducting point pattern and cluster analyses is an essential task for all field practitioners using GIS in epidemiological investigation. For a variety of reasons (explained in the handbook), most disease surveillance data are inaccessible to the public at the point or address level. Important workarounds for mapping point infor-mation in spatial epidemiological analysis include the use of kernel density estimation techniques, which often employ grid-cell methods.

It is the areal, or choropleth, mapping technique from which disease rates are derived and widely used for public consumption. The reader is guided carefully as to the issues, constraints, and procedures that require consid-eration when presenting rate outcomes in map form, including the MAUP, spatial autocorrelation, and the empirical Bayes and spatial empirical Bayes rate adjustment methods. These considerations are designed to improve the spatial–statistical strength of rate analysis and advance standardized approaches to their generation.

Spatial sampling is a key topic for leveraging the important predictive power of estimation from point observations, either from individual loca-tions or areas, to represent spatial trend in map form. This similarly employs kernel density methods, including that of geostatistics (spatial structure and measures of uncertainty), which should become part of the routine lexicon for those working in spatial epidemiology. Here the reader is familiarized with the mathematical and statistical juncture of the interpolation methods of inverse distance weighting, splines, and kriging. The mechanics of these methods, and their strengths and weaknesses, are well illustrated and will help new users to incorporate these methods into their spatial epidemiologi-cal research and maps.

In the end, the many potential uses of GIS for spatial epidemiological study are described and generate worthwhile reading for those interested in this field. The handbook also contains a sobering look at what to expect when embarking on a GIS project. Much of the effort is dependent upon sizeable startup considerations, from infrastructure to study conceptualization, data availability, and project support and management. In all, this work by our Hong Kong University colleagues is well done and a welcome addition to instructional materials emphasizing the role of geographic science in spatial epidemiology.

Charles M. Croner, Ph.D.
(*Retired February 2008*)
Centers for Disease Control and Prevention
Atlanta, Georgia

Preface

We became interested in compiling this book after having organized a few workshops and working with field epidemiologists on GIS and remote sensing applications on epidemiology and other environmental fields. There are a few academic books on spatial epidemiology covering the theoretical groundwork and statistical underpinnings of geographic variations in diseases. There are also operational guides written for specific commercial GIS software. Our book is different. In addition to the simple presentation of facts with visual examples that cater to readers with interests in geographic and spatial analyses, it also focuses on the step-by-step instructions of GIS operations based on selected freeware to encourage GIS usage in the field with a minimum cost implication on software purchase. However, we also document the more complex procedures not supported by freeware.

Mapping and GIS are important tools and methods in identifying environmental factors and possible causes of diseases. Our intent is certainly not to be exhaustive in the content coverage. Rather, we aim to provide sufficient operational detail to start the exploration process because we believe in the greater breadth of options offered by GIS and related information technologies in spatial epidemiology. Although we make general introduction to some utility functions of various freeware, the credits and intellectual rights remain with researchers and developers of these products. Throughout this book, we encourage our readers to refer to the original user manuals and sources for more in-depth discussions on the procedures and methodological context.

Our examples make use of data from two Asian regions (Thailand and Hong Kong) to illustrate the applications of GIS in examining noncontagious (asthma and dengue) and contagious (severe acute respiratory syndrome) diseases. The examples also illustrate the use of a variety of analytic approaches in studying disease incidence and patterns in different spatial scales. Geostatistical measures are also introduced to summarize patterns that are difficult to detect by examining tables of data or by visual assessment of mapped results.

We must caution readers that the information and mapping technologies that underlie GIS are constantly and rapidly changing, and it is impossible for us to keep abreast of all changes that are taking place. Although every possible effort has been made, where practicable, to check hyperlinks and ensure that the operational procedures are correct at the time of publication, some links and procedures may have changed in the interim. A simple Internet search using a part of the original Web address or by the title (or author or organization) of the original web page will generally relocate the new address. We would be remiss if we did not point out that there may be some issues more about style than about correctness in this book. None of those acknowledged is responsible for any errors the book may contain. Any errors are our sole responsibility. We would appreciate hearing from discerning readers about errors of commission or omission so that they may be addressed in future editions.

As the Chinese saying goes, experience is the mother of wisdom. We hope the GIS experience will sharpen your competitive edge and rekindle your excitement for learning.

We dedicate this book to our parents for their undivided affection and endless support over the years.*

P.C. Lai
F.M. So
K.W. Chan

*The authors declare that they have no competing interests. Use of trade names and commercial sources are for identification only and does not imply endorsement by the authors.

Acknowledgments

We thank Dr. Chuleeporn Jiraphongsa of the Ministry of Public Health of Thailand for the many opportunities to participate in the Field Epidemiology Training Programme. We are also indebted to Drs. Rungnapa Prasanthong, Pawinee Duang-ngarm, and Sopon Iamsirithaworn of the same ministry for their assistance in data preparation and collegial partnership. Our special thanks go to the Bureau of Epidemiology of Thailand for the provision of data used in our examples. We extend our sincere gratitude to Dr. Augusto Pinto of the World Health Organization for inspiring and encouraging our work in the field. Thanks also go to Dr. C.M. Wong of the Department of Community Medicine of the University of Hong Kong for involving us in health-related studies. We also acknowledge the following members of the GIS team at the Department of Geography of the University of Hong Kong for their untiring support and aspiration: Mr. Sogo S.K. Chiu, Mr. Richard K.H. Kwong, Ms. Sharon T.S. Leung, Dr. Ann A.H. Mak, and Mr. Andrew S. F. Tong.

We owe our perpetual gratitude to Prof. Gerard Rushton of the University of Iowa and Dr. Charles Croner of the U.S. CDC who wrote the forewords to this book. We much appreciate their efforts in reading the manuscript, identifying errors, and suggesting improvements.

We are grateful for the permission granted by the following researchers and organizations for the use of their products:

Prof. Luc Anselin (Spatial Analysis Laboratory, University of Illinois, Urbana-Champaign) for the use of GeoDa 0.9.5-i

Ned Levine & Associates for the use of CrimeStat III

World Health Organization for the use of the HealthMapper

ESRI for the use of ArcGIS and its extensions

We also acknowledge use of data from the following sources in Hong Kong for the preparation of the book manuscript: Census and Statistics Department, Environmental Protection Department, Department of Health, Hospital Authority, and Lands Department. Points of view or opinion contained in this book are those of the authors and do not necessarily reflect the views of the developers or agencies.

Authors

Poh-Chin Lai has been an associate professor in the Department of Geography of the University of Hong Kong since 1993 and honorary deputy director of the Geographical/Land Information System Research Centre of the same university. She was also the associate dean of the Faculty of Arts from 1998 to 2003. She obtained her doctorate degree in computer cartography in 1983 from the University of Waterloo in Ontario, Canada. Before joining the University of Hong Kong, she was affiliated with the Department of Geodetic Science and Surveying of The Ohio State University from 1989 to 1992 and the Department of Geography of the University of Maryland in College Park from 1983 to 1989. Dr. Lai specializes in digital cartography and GISs and has served as a technical consultant to various public, government, and international agencies. Her current research interests entail use of the geospatial technologies (including geographic information, remote sensing, cartographic and geostatistical analyses) in a diverse range of public and environmental health issues. Her co-edited book entitled *GIS for Health and the Environment: Development in the Asia-Pacific Region* was released in July 2007 by Springer-Verlag.

Fun-Mun So is a senior GIS consultant having extensive and hands-on experience in providing a wide range of GIS solutions and project management for government organizations and the business sector. He obtained his master of philosophy degree from the University of Hong Kong and has since engaged in IT solutions, systems design and migration, and GIS application development. His research interests cover geo-demographic segmentation or profiling, geographic data alignment, disease and environmental associative analysis, and geostatistics. He is also active in GIS training programs in school education, environmental assessment, and spatial analysis in human disease surveillance. His latest publications involve studies about the spatial association between respiratory diseases and air pollution.

Ka-Wing Chan is a GIS specialist experienced in curriculum development, disease mapping, and spatial analysis of crime. She is presently the assistant program coordinator of the Taught Master GIS program at the University of Hong Kong. She gained her master of philosophy degree in GISs in 2003. Her thesis, entitled "A GIS Approach to the Spatial Analysis of Crime in Urban Areas: A Case Study of Mongkok, Hong Kong," won the Best MPhil Research Award 2003–2005 from the Hong Kong Geographic Information Systems Association. She is co-authoring with P.C. Lai and Ann S.H. Mak in developing teaching materials for the new secondary geography GIS curriculum and has participated in various projects, including the spatial analysis of SARS and childhood obesity in Hong Kong, as well as estimating population size in emergency situations using spatial interpolation techniques.

List of Acronyms

Refer to the *AGI GIS Dictionary* (www.geo.ed.ac.uk/agidict/alpha.html) for an explanation of the various terminologies. It contains numerous terms that either relate directly to GIS or which GIS users may encounter.

AIDS Acquired immune deficiency syndrome
API Air pollution index
ASCII American Standard Code for Information Interchange
CDC Centers for Disease Control and Prevention
CPU Central processing unit
DAT File format of MapInfo
DBF Proprietary file format of dBase III/IV/V
DBMS Database management system
DC District councils, a census enumeration unit of Hong Kong and formerly known as District Boards
DCCA District council constituency areas, a census enumeration unit of Hong Kong
EDA Electronic design automation
GIS Geographic information systems
GML Geography markup language
GPS Global Positioning Systems
HIV Human immunodeficiency virus
HTML Hypertext markup language
HTTP Hypertext transfer protocol
ICD International Classification of Diseases is the classification code for mortality data from death certificates. In Hong Kong, the International Classification of Diseases, Clinical Modification (ICD-9-CM) is used to code and classify morbidity data from inpatient and outpatient records.
IDW Inverse distance weighted
KML Keyhole markup language for managing 3D geospatial data in Google Earth and Google Maps
LISA Local indicators of spatial association
LSBG Large street block geographic (boundary)
MAUP Modifiable areal unit problem
MDB File format of Microsoft Access
MHz Megahertz
NNI Nearest neighbor index
NOAA National Oceanic and Atmospheric Administration (United States)
OCR Optical character recognition
ODBC Open database connectivity
PC Personal computer

PDA   Personal digital assistant
RAM   Random-access memory
RS   Remote sensing
SBR   Standardized morbidity ratio
SBU   Street block planning unit, a census enumeration unit of Hong Kong
SDE   Standard deviational ellipse
SHP   Proprietary file format of ESRI's line of products
SMR   Standardized mortality ratio
SPU   Secondary planning unit, a census enumeration unit of Hong Kong
STI   Sexually transmitted infections
TIGER Topologically Integrated Geographic Encoding and Referencing
TIN   Triangulated irregular network
TPU   Tertiary planning unit, a census enumeration unit of Hong Kong
WHO   World Health Organization
XML   Extensible markup language

1

GIS Concepts and Operations

1.1 What Is a GIS?

GIS is an acronym for geographic information science, or geographic information studies, or geographic information systems. Whereas the term *science* is used to connote basic research and *studies* is associated with education-related undertakings, *systems* is adopted mostly for the applied situations. Indeed, a GIS is a computerized setting whose information management functions are comparable to those of a banking information system for handling transactions of financial accounts. It is also compatible with a library information system that gathers, creates, stores, processes, and retrieves catalogs of books and references. However, unlike information systems driven mainly by alphanumeric data entries, a GIS has a distinct component of geography or location that captures and represents features on the surface of the Earth (Figure 1.1). These geographic features are more widely known as georeferenced or spatial data.

The question "what is a GIS?" has been asked and answered by many. Burrough[1] provided a toolbox-based definition that a GIS is "a powerful set of tools for collecting, storing, retrieving, transforming and displaying spatial data from the real world." Smith et al.[2] purported a data-based definition and viewed GIS as "a database system in which most of the data are spatially indexed, and upon which a set of procedures operated in order to answer queries about spatial entities in the database." Cowen[3] subsequently suggested an organization-based definition, stating that GIS is "a decision support system involving the integration of spatially referenced data in a problem solving environment."

Whichever is the preferred definition, a GIS is generally seen as a customizable digital computer-based platform whose generic functions are designed to work with geographic data to perform multifaceted and multipurpose tasks.[4] The multiplicity and adaptability of GIS has meant that there are common and sharable functionalities across many disciplines. The use of GIS in public health and spatial epidemiology is but one example. The use of GIS in any field requires a strong knowledge base of both the tool and the science. This apparent dual requirement in using GIS has resulted in a growing demand for interdisciplinary teamwork and improved scientific usability in

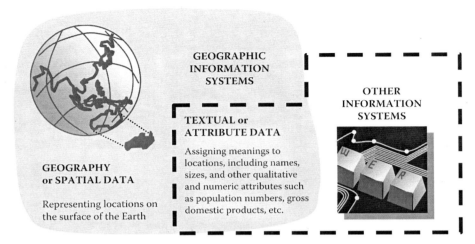

FIGURE 1.1
GIS versus other information systems.

many nontraditional settings (such as public participatory planning, community emergency preparedness and response, and other activities). In short, these qualities of a GIS environment offer an exciting opportunity to develop the role and science of geography and many other fields of interest and study.

The focus of this book concerns the basic approaches and use of GIS in spatial epidemiology. *Spatial epidemiology* is defined by Elliot and Wartenberg[5] as "the description and analysis of geographically indexed health data with respect to demographic, environmental, behavioral, socioeconomic, genetic, and infectious risk factors." Waller and Gotway[6] defined spatial epidemiology as "a dynamic body of theory and analytic methods concerned with the study of spatial patterns of disease incidence and mortality." They also suggested that an increased recognition of maps as a useful tool in illuminating potential causes of a disease has sparked interest in spatial epidemiology. As much as possible, our examples make use of public domain GIS as opposed to commercially available GIS platforms, which have been widely discussed.

1.2   What a GIS Is Not

A GIS is not merely a mapmaking tool, although mapping and spatial queries are its two main activities. Maps are often a product of the system because they offer a better way to visualize the results from spatial analyses. A GIS is also not simply a software package because software is only one of its many collective components, which are discussed in the following section. Besides, it is different from a conventional information system with dedicated functions just for the manipulation and query of alphanumeric data because a GIS has additional capabilities for spatial data analysis and visualization.

The spatial analytical power of a GIS is uniquely different from the capabilities expected of a map, a software package, or a numerical information system. Spatial analysis concerns the questions about "what phenomena are where" and "where things are in relation to each other." Data stored in a GIS are not simply maps but a spatial database that combines attribute and spatial data with a dynamic linkage between them. The system offers a method for collecting, manipulating, analyzing, and displaying geographic data and their concordant relationships both in space and over time. Maps in a GIS are a graphic representation of one or more digital databases that interactively can produce new views for improved understanding in analysis. A GIS also allows the user to integrate data from a variety of sources or formats, in particular, by layering the data such that queries, selections, and various investigative procedures can act on the spatial and attribute data therein.

1.3   GIS Components and Functionalities

A GIS uses geographically referenced and nonspatial data and includes operations that support spatial analysis. According to *A Practitioner's Guide to GIS Terminology*, spatial analysis is the process of extracting or creating new information about a set of geographic features to perform routine examination, assessment, evaluation, analysis, or modeling of data in a geographic area based on preestablished and computerized criteria and standards.[7] The connection between elements of a GIS is geography (i.e., location, proximity, and spatial distribution) (Figure 1.2). A GIS is also an enabling technology because of the potential it offers for a wide variety of disciplines that depend on spatial information.

GIS has two key activities: (1) to visualize spatial information, or "make maps," and (2) to analyze spatial information, or "ask questions of the maps and data." Through these activities, the user gains a better understanding of the geographic phenomenon being studied — to know where things are, see patterns, find relationships, query geographic characteristics, monitor changes, and link observations with research. To enable geographic exploration with a computer, spatial data must be structured and encoded in a specific manner (discussed in the next chapter).

The consensus based on the definitions offered by various scholars is that a GIS has five major components: data, equipment (including both hardware and software), methods (including models and operational rules), people, and organization (Figure 1.3).[8] Spatial data, which must reside in some sort of a

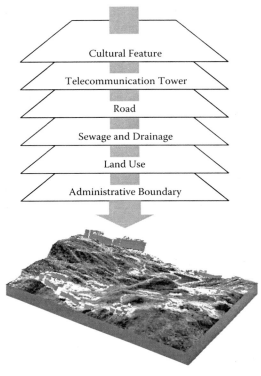

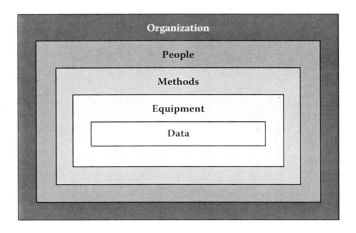

FIGURE 1.2
Connection between elements of a GIS is geography.

FIGURE 1.3
Components of a GIS.

hardware platform and be accessible via software, are at the heart of a GIS. In addition, the data must be structured according to several models, and their organization, retrieval, and manipulation are governed by operational rules. Skilled personnel are needed to operate the system and process the spatial data. More important, the GIS operation must function within an organizational or institutional setting with specific scopes and mission statements.

1.3.1 Data

In terms of GIS applications in spatial epidemiology, the locations of the cohort population (where they are, or the spatial component) and their characteristics (what they are about, or the attributes) are the bases for further spatial analysis. Compared to a decade ago, digital data have become more affordable and widely available. The most widely available spatial data are remotely sensed, especially satellite imageries, and paper maps (Figure 1.4). Although a number of government, international, and private agencies are offering secondary data in digital or printed formats for purchase or free downloads over the Internet, there is a growing demand for spatial databases for dedicated use through field data collection techniques.

The importance of GIS data and the structural arrangement for digital processing cannot be overemphasized. Chapter 2 offers a detailed account of the characteristics of geographic data, their sources, and representational models for space–time analysis. Techniques for data capture and conversion are also discussed.

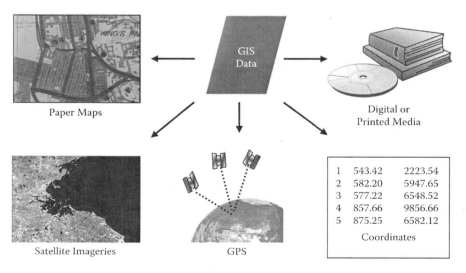

FIGURE 1.4
Types of GIS data.

1.3.2 Equipment

A GIS cannot operate without a prescribed hardware and software setup. Today, GIS is no longer restricted to function only on high-end workstations. Indeed, it has become more widely used in a Windows-based desktop on PCs (Figure 1.5). The trend is moving toward portable and mobile devices for on-demand or real-time spatial processing of data.

Most GIS operations can be accommodated with a minimum systems configuration of the Windows-compatible setting, 200-MHz PC processor, and 128-MB RAM. In general, a faster system is preferred because some GIS operations are CPU-intensive and require substantial disk space. Given that maps and graphic visualization are key functions of a GIS, the RAM and video RAM in particular should be maximized to ensure smoother and seamless operations that enable dynamic visual displays. Peripheral devices such as GPS or video camera also are available to support spatial data input and output operations (Figure 1.6). The acquisition of these devices must be factored into any operational GIS setup to allow for flexibility in creating in-house data and customizing output.

A range of GIS software is available, either for purchase or for download, in the market (see Appendix A). The choice of GIS software hinges on various selection criteria, including functional requirements, ease of use, and cost, but should be tailored to the needs of the individual or the agency. Although some criteria require expert advice, the matter of cost is, unfortunately, more tangible and can often become the overriding factor in a GIS implementation. An important trend has been the increasing availability of GIS shareware for free downloads over the Internet (see Appendix A and Chapters 4 through 6). These shareware are often crafted for specific purposes and contain a subset of functions either specially designed for those purposes or extracted from a full-scale GIS. Also, some freeware may contain functions unique to an application domain that are not available in GIS software catered for generic purposes. Whether commercial or shareware, it is highly desirable to acquire GIS software that supports interoperability and conforms to open-source standards such as XML- and GML-coded interfaces.[9]

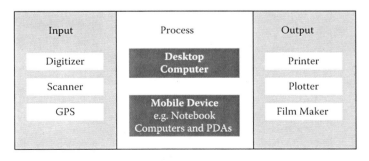

FIGURE 1.5
Hardware configurations for GIS operations.

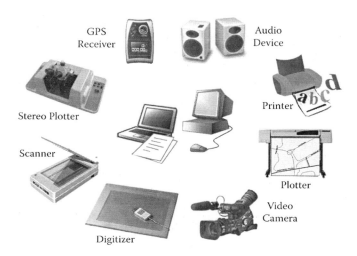

FIGURE 1.6
Peripheral devices for GIS operation.

1.3.3 Methods

Methods often imply the manner of encoding geographic data for GIS processing (which are elaborated on in Chapters 2 and 3). A broader explanation encompasses familiarity with the operational procedures of a GIS, program algorithms, substance- or content-specific knowledge, spatial analytical skills, and cartographic techniques. These matters will be discussed in the context of spatial epidemiology and illustrated in subsequent chapters. It suffices to say that the essence of this book is about methods in dealing with epidemiological data from the spatial perspective.

1.3.4 People

Given the range of GIS technical and knowledge skills, there is no doubt that teamwork is an essential requirement in a GIS setting. The most crucial requirement of a successful GIS operation is having well-trained personnel and thinking operators. Although these are self-taught individuals, most of them acquire operational skills either from on-the-job training or through vendor-specific training programs. An increasing number of formal academic curricula (including "GIS certification"), usually based on one to two years of specialized study, are now available.

GIS users in general can be categorized according to their level of content knowledge and technical proficiency (Figure 1.7). The term technologists implies a group of users with a moderate level of technical skills but more characterized with an advanced understanding of the application areas. This group of users is not large in number and represents managers or administrators in charge of GIS operations. They are often the key personnel who craft,

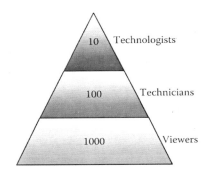

FIGURE 1.7
A conceptual framework of GIS user skills.

design, and set up the GIS operations and deal with the daily process and flow of information, including data quality and validation decisions.

Technicians in the middle tier comprise individuals with a high level of proficiency in technical and operational expertise. This group is larger in number and is the key to the successful execution of GIS tasks. These individuals may not have full knowledge of the entire application environment but can deliver results using a GIS. The group includes programmers who execute operational requirements and procedures to allow the group of less technical users (indicated at the base tier of Figure 1.7) to view and use the results. The viewers at the base level, however, may include decision makers of an organization who need access to results and information of a GIS but do not have the time to learn and master the operational procedures.

We have presented a conceptualization of a GIS personnel structure for an organization. In practice, GIS is sustainable only with an effective plan of personnel deployment within an organization and suitable retraining programs.

1.3.5 Organization

GIS has proliferated in the West because its adoption has mostly taken the bottom-up approach, whereas the top-down course from the state or government is more evident in the East, particularly in Asian countries. Almost without exception, an organizational setting with the technical viabilities and champion advocates is key to the adoption of GIS technology.[10] Also, it is evident that the widespread utility of GIS hinges on the availability of digital spatial data (often produced by government sources) that are offered as public domain products at nominal or recoverable costs.

Organizational support is instrumental to achieving and maintaining GIS implementation. Organizations need to consider policies on data acquisition, standards, interoperability, and sharing, all of which influence the efficiency of daily GIS operations. The single most important obstacle against the widespread adoption of GIS methods in many developing countries has been a shortage of affordable and updated data.

In summary, GIS usage can be evaluated by a multitude of measures including speed of data entry and integration, range or robustness of functionality, ease of use, and data volume or capacity for different applications and users (Figure 1.8). The compilation of digital data for GIS operations can be costly and time consuming, whereas the methods of integration can become complex for certain data types. The procurement of equipment to

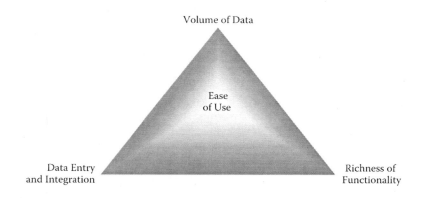

FIGURE 1.8
Concerns for GIS performance.

accommodate capacity is comparatively straightforward, although personnel and skill requirements are often underestimated. Organizational problems, however, may be the most complex because they encompass interagency and intraagency relations and technical complications.

1.4   Basic GIS Operations

GIS offers a platform to bring together all types of data based on geographic identifiers or Earth location (e.g., latitude and longitude). Like many other information systems, a GIS embodies operations for data input, process, and output. Figure 1.9 illustrates, in greater detail, these functions within a GIS. The categorization is somewhat arbitrary and not mutually exclusive. Although some of the functions (e.g., display and query of the database) are found in all three stages of a GIS operation, those functions on the left relate more to data input and those on the right for routine data output. Spatial analysis tools (at the bottom) in general are associated with a higher level of data processing requirements and are the focus of this book.

Data creation and editing concern the acquisition of both spatial and non-spatial (attribute) data. Procedures include entry and update of coordinate and attribute data that may need to be processed further to conform to data standards or structures. The structuring process may involve simple transformation of nominal geographic identifiers, map projections, registration of coordinate data, and conversion between various data structures or formats. Besides quality assurance, the purpose of these procedures is to ascertain compatibility among different data coverages and scales. These procedures are a crucial preparation for subsequent spatial data analysis.

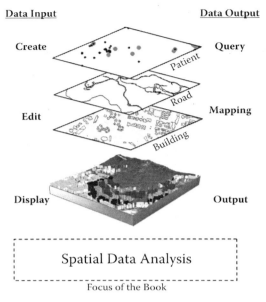

FIGURE 1.9
Basic GIS functionality.

GIS processes embrace a variety of spatial analyses covering a range of modeling possibilities (natural resources, urban and built environments, retail establishments, transport flows, and diffusion) and visualization (mapping, three- or higher-dimensional, and space–time animation) procedures. Included are tools for visual displays, database queries, and single- and multiple-layer operations. Four traditional types of spatial analysis can be identified: (1) spatial overlay and contiguity analysis (Figure 1.10a), (2) surface or multidimensional analysis (Figure 1.10b), (3) linear or network analysis (Figure 1.10c), and (4) raster- or grid-based analysis (Figure 1.10d). Some GIS functions for spatial analysis include the following: neighborhood or buffer operations, Thiessen polygons, Boolean functions of union and intersect, shortest-path routing, location and allocation functions, and surface or terrain modeling. These methods will be examined in subsequent chapters.

Data output and presentation entail visual displays as well as the design and preparation of maps and written outputs. Besides functions for tabular layout and report form generation, GIS functions for this category also offer cartographic and thematic mapping, charting, and drafting support tools for map composition. Although maps and summary tables are a powerful presentation of results from spatial analysis, what must be remembered is that the conclusions drawn should be interpreted in light of other information, including knowledge about the phenomenon under study and the local context.

There are limitations and caveats to the use of GIS techniques in epidemiology and outbreak investigation. The mapping of diseases tends to expose the "where" but not necessarily the "why there" of an outbreak.[11] Nevertheless,

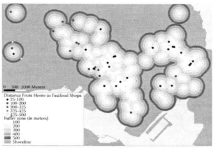

(a) Spatial Overlay and Contiguity Analysis

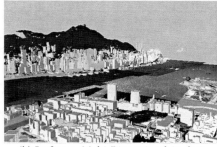

(b) Surface or Multi-Dimensional Analysis

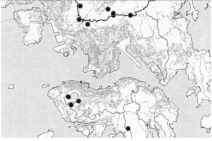

(c) Linear or Network Analysis

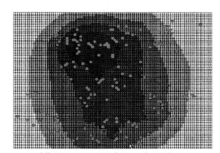

(d) Raster or Grid-Based Analysis

FIGURE 1.10
A color version of this figure follows page 108 Types of spatial data analysis: (a) spatial overlay and contiguity analysis, (b) surface or multidimensional analysis, (c) linear or network analysis, and (d) raster- or grid-based analysis.

disease mapping can offer new insights into areas of concern and, importantly, be a source of new hypotheses and research design for further exploratory analyses. Not only can map patterns provide stimuli for generating new possibilities underlying disease causation[12,13] but they also can promote the use of other investigative tools in outbreak control (such as CrimeStat), as will be illustrated throughout the remainder of this book.

1.5 Summary

This introductory chapter offers a brief overview of GIS and a description of its basic functionality. Chapter 2 focuses on GIS input operations, whereas the means of undertaking and visualizing spatial analyses are explored in subsequent chapters. A number of spatial analytical methods are discussed in Chapters 3 through 6 with reference to the two key activities of GIS: (1) to visualize spatial information, or "make maps," and (2) to analyze spatial information, or "ask questions of the maps and data." These activities are used in elementary, cluster, and contextual analyses referred to by Bailey and Gatrell.[14] Elementary analysis involves the making of maps to allow simple visual inspection of a geographic phenomenon. Cluster analysis attempts to identify possible spatial distributional patterns (whether clustered, dispersed, or random). Contextual analysis aims at explaining relationships between geographic phenomena (whether there is spatial autocorrelation) or temporal variations (whether there is a space–time trend). In some GIS modeling procedures, prediction can be made with reference to existing trends and distributional patterns. Procedures to adopt the GIS approach in epidemiological studies are summarized in Chapter 7. This book closes with a chapter documenting the developments and evolutions of GIS with a note of caution about its applications. GIS is a tool for integrating thinkers. With practice, anyone can learn how to execute GIS data operational functions, but to adapt GIS to an application setting and apply it wisely is a more elusive skill.

References

1. Burrough, P.A., Principles of Geographic Information Systems for Land Assessment, Oxford University Press, New York, NY, 1986.
2. Smith, T.R., Menon, S., Starr, J.L., and Estes, J.E., Requirements and principles for the implementation and construction of large-scale geographic information systems, *International Journal of Geographical Information Systems*, 1, 13, 1987.
3. Cowen, D.J., GIS versus CAD versus DBMS: what are the differences?, *Photogrammetric Engineering and Remote Sensing*, 54, 1551, 1988.
4. Longley, P.A., Goodchild, M.F., Maguire, D.J., and Rhind D.W., *Geographic Information Systems and Science*, 2nd ed., Wiley, Hoboken, NJ, 2005.
5. Elliot, P., and Wartenberg, D., Spatial epidemiology: current approaches and future challenges, *Environmental Health Perspectives*, 112(9), 998, 2004.
6. Waller, L.A., and Gotway, C.A., *Applied Spatial Statistics for Public Health Data*, Wiley, Hoboken, NJ, 2004.
7. Wood, S.J., *A Practitioner's Guide to GIS Terminology: A Glossary of Geographic Information System Terms*, Data West Research Agency, University Place, WA, 2000. Available: http://www.geocities.com/gisdatawest [accessed on June 10, 2006].
8. Goodchild, M.F., What is geographic information science?, *NCGIA Core Curriculum in GIScience*, October 7, 1997. Available: http://www.ncgia.ucsb.edu/giscc/units/u002/u002.html [accessed on June 10, 2006].
9. Croner, C.M., Public health, GIS, and the Internet, *Annual Reviews of Public Health*, 24, 51, 2003. Available: http://www.cdc.gov/nchs/data/gis/GIS_AND_THE_INTERNET.pdf [accessed on October 15, 2007].
10. Nebraska Geographic Information Systems Steering Committee, Planning a successful GIS implementation (*draft*), *Nebraska Guidebook for a Local Government Multipurpose Land Information System*, VIII-1. Available: http://www.calmit.unl.edu/gis/LIS_Imp_Plan_4-25.pdf [accessed on June 10, 2006].

11. Howe, G.M., National Atlas of Disease Mortality in the United Kingdom, T. Nelson, London, 1963.

12. McKee, K.T., Jr., Shields, T.M., Jenkins, P.R., Zenilman, J.M., and Glass, G.E., Application of a geographic information system to the tracking and control of an outbreak of shigellosis. *Clinical Infectious Diseases*, 31(3), 728, 2000.

13. Lloyd, O.L., and Yu, T.S., Disease mapping: a valuable technique for environmental medicine. *Journal of Hong Kong Medical Association*, 46(1), 3, 1994.

14. Bailey, T.C., and Gatrell, A.C., *Interactive Spatial Data Analysis*, Longman, Essex, 1995.

2

GIS and Geographic Data

2.1 Characteristics of Geographic Data

Geographic data are inherently a form of spatial data because they concern the physical dimension and have a spatial location in the real world.[1] These data tell us information about our world, and their locations are defined by using Earth-based locational coordinate referencing systems. Two common systems of coordinate georeferencing are the spherical and Cartesian systems (Figure 2.1). The spherical coordinate system describes a position on the surface of the Earth in terms of a pair of readings in northing (parallel or latitude) and easting (meridian or longitude). The latitudes (y coordinates) range from 0° to 90° in the northern hemisphere, starting at the equator and moving toward the North Pole. Similarly, the values range from 0° to −90° in the southern hemisphere, moving from the equator to the South Pole. The longitudes (x coordinates) range from 0° to +180° in the eastern hemisphere, starting at the prime meridian in Greenwich, England, and traveling eastward across Europe, Africa, and Asia. The range in the western hemisphere, also beginning at the prime meridian but traveling westward across the American continents, is from 0° to −180°.

The Cartesian coordinate system is also called the planar or plane coordinate system. It is a local measurement system created in association with a map projection[2] and describes locations in terms of distances or angles from a fixed reference point. All positions have two values (x and y) measured in reference to the origin (0, 0). The x coordinate is the horizontal position, and the y coordinate is the vertical position. Measurements of length, area, and angle are in constant units across the two dimensions.

The examples in subsequent chapters make use of data from two geographic regions of different sizes: Thailand and Hong Kong (Figure 2.2). Thailand is situated in Southeast Asia and shares its border with Myanmar in the west and north, Laos in the northeast, Cambodia in the east, and Malaysia in the south. It covers an area of 514,000 km2 extending about 1,700 km in the north–south direction and 800 km in the east–west direction. Hong Kong is a small territory comprising a group of islands and peninsula at the mouth of the Pearl River. It has a land area of 1,078 km2, extending about 40 km in the north–south direction and 60 km in the east–west direction. Both

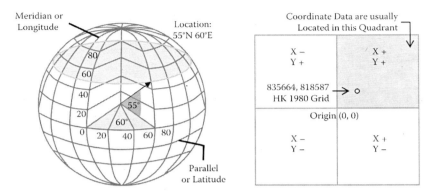

FIGURE 2.1
Spherical (left) and Cartesian (right) coordinate systems.

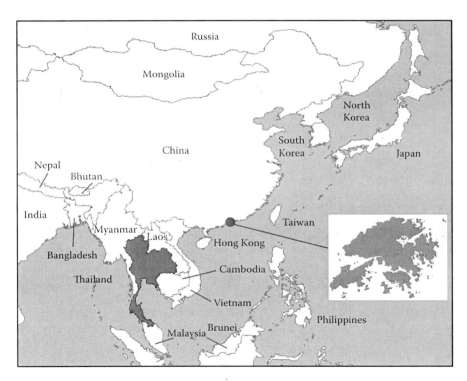

FIGURE 2.2
A map of South Asia showing Thailand and Hong Kong.

regions use the Universal Transverse Mercator (UTM) map projection, which maintains shape and is commonly used to portray larger areas with more extensive north–south than east–west extent. Thailand lies in the UTM projection zone 47N, with elevation in meters above sea level. Hong Kong uses the HK1980 grid, which is the local plane coordinate system modified from the UTM, with an origin situated southwest of Lantau Island and adding 800,000 m to its northings and eastings.

2.1.1 Topological Relations

Geographic data have two component parts: spatial and nonspatial (Figure 2.3). Spatial data contain locational information and are recorded by geometry. They form the basis for drawing maps. Nonspatial data contain

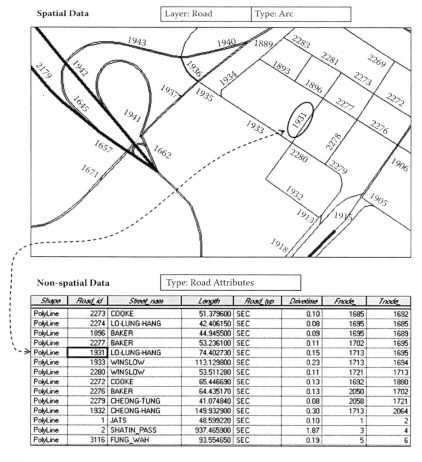

FIGURE 2.3
Spatial data are related to nonspatial data by a unique identifier.

descriptive information about the spatial features represented. They are stored as rows of entries in digital computerized attribute tables. The columns of items store descriptive or quantitative attributes for each spatial feature. Spatial data are related to nonspatial data via a unique identifier that exists in both the spatial and attribute domains.

Topology is defined as the neighborhood relationships[3] and concerns the relative positioning of spatial features. In many geographic applications of social interaction, the relative positioning among features or activities is more significant than the absolute positioning of acute accuracy. For example, it makes more sense in vehicle navigation to know the relative location of an approaching destination (e.g., whether a hospital is to the left or right side of a road) than its actual address or coordinates. Furthermore, some locations (e.g., possible areas of disease risks) do not have clearly defined boundaries and are often "described" with reference to some known locations (e.g., in the vicinity of a housing estate or a community). The definition of an area, and thus its boundary, in many health and disease applications is not clearly defined and may not conform to or align with census enumeration or other administrative units.

Topology is fundamental to GIS geographic and map analysis and its underlying spatial search and query operations. Three types of topological relations are either explicitly or implicitly coded in geographic data: connectivity, adjacency, and containment (Figure 2.4). Connectivity describes the "from–to" relationship, typically for point-to-point travel along a route or to show direct and indirect linkages between places. Adjacency expresses the "next-to" or "border-on" relationship as exemplified by adjoining areas. Containment pictures the "located in/on" or "belong-to" relationships to indicate if an area is enclosed by another. The presence of these topological relations is the key to enabling spatial queries and analyses of epidemiological observations with other geographic features or objects.

Topology	Spatial Epidemiological Queries
Connectivity • From/to	➤ Find the nearest hospital and how to get there!
Adjacency • Next to • Borders on	➤ Estimate the total number of households within 5 m (borders on) and 5–20 m (next to) of an infected building.
Containment • Located in/on • Belongs to	➤ How many persons within a district are infected? ➤ To which residential district does this infected person belong?

FIGURE 2.4
Topological relations in spatial queries.

2.2 GIS Models: Raster versus Vector

As illustrated in Figure 2.3, attribute data contain alphanumeric contents and are organized in a tabular structure with rows of records and columns of items. This structure is quite common and comparatively easy to handle in a DBMS. Spatial or mapped data, however, present a uniquely different situation. Putting aside the matter of map scale (whether global or local) and coordinate referencing (whether spherical or Cartesian), the cartographic elements from a variety of sources, as illustrated in Figure 1.4 of Chapter 1, must first be encoded and structured for digital processing.

In general, two classes of models have been established to handle spatial data. Broadly speaking, the vector model symbolizes spatial data as point, line, or area features, whereas the raster model reduces spatial data into a series of grid cells[1] (Figure 2.5). The two models can coexist and are inter-changeable in most GIS, with the vector model preferred for local scale operations and the raster model for regional or global scale applications. The vector model has the advantage of bearing more detailed encoding or being more "intelligent" but is more resource-intensive in its preparation. The raster model has the advantage of attaining an extensive coverage but lacks explicit detail in its encoded representation unless it goes through image interpretation and analysis.

Reality – an Aerial Photograph

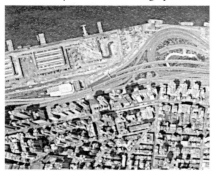

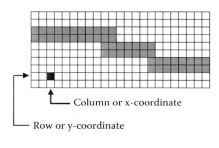

Column or x-coordinate

Row or y-coordinate

Raster uses Square Cells to Model Reality

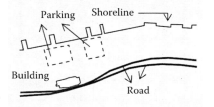

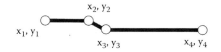

Vector Makes Discrete Representations of Features in Reality

FIGURE 2.5
Vector and raster data models.

Although the two models are interchangeable for the most part, care must be taken to ensure that the scale of operation, data resolution, and application domain are compatible. Combining data from different periods, varying map scales, and nonstandardized data classifications will invariably introduce errors, some of which may significantly affect analytical results.

As indicated earlier, geographic data have two component parts: spatial (locational) and aspatial (attribute). A number of formats are available to encode spatial data in the vector or raster models — a result of the many selections of hardware and software platforms that have evolved throughout the development history of GIS and information technologies (Table 2.1). The aspatial data are also processed via various spreadsheet or database tools into different storage formats.

TABLE 2.1
Popular Formats of GIS Data Processing

Format	Remarks
Vector	
DLG	Digital line graph, a data transfer format by the U.S. Geological survey
DWG	An undocumented and proprietary native binary format for drawing files created by AutoCAD
DXF	Drawing interchange or exchange format for Autodesk's AutoCAD
E00	Arc/Info export file for data interchange
GML	Geography markup language, XML standard for exchanging and saving geographic vector data
MIF/MID	MapInfo interchange format
SHP	ESRI shapefile
SIF	Standard intergraph format for intergraph systems
SVG	Scalable vector graphics
TIGER	Topologically Integrated Geographic Encoding and Referencing by the U.S. Census Bureau
VXP	Idrisi32 ASCII Vector export format
WMF	Microsoft Windows metafile
Raster	
AVHRR	Advanced very high resolution radiometer file; NOAA satellite data
BMP	Bitmap format
DEM	Digital elevation model, a raster format used by the U.S. Geological Survey to store elevation information
EPS	Encapsulated PostScript
GeoTIFF	Geographic Tagged Image File Format of Landsat and QuickBird images; this format is supported by Photoshop and most GIS software
GIF	Graphics interchange format
IMG	Raster data format of ERDAS IMAGINE
JERS-1	Japanese Earth Resource Satellite–1
JPG or JPEG	Joint Photographic Experts Group file format for images and photographs on Web pages

TABLE 2.1 (continued)
Popular Formats of GIS Data Processing

Format	Remarks
Landsat Thematic Mapper (TM)	Format for imageries from the LANDSAT satellite by the U.S.
PCX	A common raster format produced by most scanners and PC drawing programs
SPOT	Imageries from the SPOT satellite by France come in DIMAP (digital image MAP in mid-2002 for SPOT 5 satellite) or CAP (format for SPOT Scene products developed by the Centre d'Archivage et de Prétraitement) formats
TIF or TIFF	Tagged Image File Format for storing high-resolution bit-mapped, gray-scale, and color images
Yaogan II	China's new remote sensing satellite; can export files in GeoTIFF and TIFF formats
Attribute	
ASCII	American Standard Code for Information Interchange
DBF	Aston-Tate dBase DBMS file format
MDB	Microsoft Access database file format
FMB or FMT	Oracle file format
XLS	Microsoft Excel worksheet format
123	Lotus 123 97 file format
TXT	Text format

The existence of many commercial and public domain utility programs for GIS and data processing brings about the format problems of geographic data. The commercial products, in particular, come with proprietary formats of some variation from the industry standards and hinder, to a certain extent, casual and crossover use among the products. The proliferation of these computer wares in the market has necessitated data transfer standards to facilitate the exchange of data between different GIS systems and computer platforms. Nowadays, a data format can be exported into other popular data formats, and a GIS can also allow imports of selected data formats other than its own. The following discussions pertain to some of the more commonly used formats of geographic data.

2.2.1 Raster

Raster data are grid-based data that are most frequently used for recording images (e.g., photographs, satellite scenes). Aerial photographs are early versions of pictorial representation of the Earth's surface. Nowadays, remotely sensed and multispectral images of the Earth's surface (e.g., Landsat, SPOT, JERS, QuickBird) through sophisticated sensors mounted on satellites have become popular for mapping areas with extensive ground coverage.

Raster data registered in various formats (BMP, GIF, JPG, etc.) contain grid cells encoded in different gray tones or colors. The size of the grid cells is kept uniform for an image and corresponds to an area on the ground; the larger the ground coverage, the lower the resolution (e.g., 30×30 Km^2 is of a lower resolution compared with 10×10 Km^2). The images must be georeferenced to the same coordinate system to stack on top of each other, and superimposing images of varying resolution can be tricky. Aerial photographs and remotely sensed imageries in the raster formats can be further analyzed by examining the spectral bands through digital image processing techniques.[4]

2.2.2 Vector

There are many variations of the vector format differentiated largely by the organization of the internal component files. The vector data model of the arc–node format is the most representative. The digital line graph (DLG) and TIGER structures (developed by the U.S. Geological Survey and the Bureau of Census, respectively) are pioneers in this form of spatial data representation. In this model, geographic features are scale-dependent and are reduced to point, line, and area objects. Although most features can be symbolized by one of three representations as points, lines, or areas, certain complex features may have a mix of representations at the same scale. For example, a river can be characterized as an area feature near its mouth but with its tributaries presented as lines. Likewise, larger cities are drawn as area features and smaller towns marked as points.

Perhaps the most apparent difference between raster and vector representation lies in their methods of data capture. A raster map can be created by the relatively effortless scanning process, but a vector map must be digitized (i.e., tracing each point, line, and area featured on a printed map) by manual or semiautomated means. The raster representation is thus less resource-intensive in its preparation, but the vector data are more "intelligent" given their detailed encapsulation of topological relations.

2.2.3 Attribute

Attribute data are alphanumeric in value and prepared in the same way as other text-based files. The ready availability of spreadsheet programs and database systems has made the organization and editing of textual data convenient. Textual data on printed pages also may be scanned with an optical character recognition (OCR) program for direct conversion into the digital representation. These digital tabular entries can be imported straight into a GIS to combine with their respective spatial data through a column of unique identifiers common to both, as illustrated in Figure 2.3.

2.3 Data for Spatial Epidemiological Studies

Based on the preceding discussions, we note that there are many types of data in different formats. A spatial epidemiological study will likely make use of these data to varying degrees. Two types of data are needed: disease (essential) and spatial (additional) (Table 2.2). The essential data provide the geographic context upon which to plot disease cases for visualization. The additional data on environmental or sociodemographic characteristics are needed to either augment visualization or support more in-depth analysis of the disease or health outcome.

Elliott et al.[5] advised that the ideal data for spatial epidemiological research would consist of information on the population of a study area such as their individual characteristics, movements, personal exposures, and subsequent health records. However, it was recognized that a considerable investment in time and resources was required to obtain such a comprehensive data set. In most cases, three sources of disease data are available: those from hospital discharges, mortality and morbidity records, and surveillance or independent research.

Hospital discharge records offer a rich source of information about the patterns of care, the public health burden, injury morbidity, and costs associated with chronic diseases. These data can be used to identify public health priorities for a more focused public health program, as well as gaining the attention of policy makers. Patient data often incorporated in hospital discharge records include gender, age (date of birth), residential address, postal code, disease diagnosis code, and admission and discharge dates of an epi-

TABLE 2.2

Types of Data Used in Spatial Epidemiological Studies

Essential Data	Description
1a. Health or disease	Vital statistics, notifiable diseases, patient registries, and health surveys from various international or government agencies [Note: Address data must be geocoded to obtain spatial referencing.]
1b. Field epidemiology	Surveyed data on disease occurrences with location coordinates collected with a GPS
2a. Spatially referenced base	Digital cartographic data available from various international or government agencies [Note: Usually of topographic nature to include contours, rivers, and features of a built environment]
Additional Data	**Description**
2b. Remotely sensed	Land cover, elevation, soil type as reflected by satellite imageries
2c. Environmental and natural resources	Interpreted data on land use, water quality, air quality, climate, geology, etc.
3. Census or demographic	Sociodemographic and economic data aggregated by some enumeration areas

sode. These data are important for conducting epidemiological studies of disease etiology.

Mortality data on individuals are obtainable from the death registry of most immigration departments. Like most developed countries where death is well-recorded, Hong Kong has maintained since 1995 a detailed account of the number of deaths from each disease in statistical reports published annually by the Hospital Authority.[6] The contents include gender, age, and cause and place of death but not the individual's residential address in order to maintain confidentiality. The method for estimating the morbidity of a disease is more complicated than that of mortality.[7–9] *Morbidity* is defined as the incidence of a disease within a population. While *incidence* refers to the number of new cases of a disease being diagnosed or reported for a population during a defined period, *prevalence* refers to the number of people in a population with a disease at a particular time, regardless of when the illness began. By definition, the prevalence rate is more appropriate if we wish to know how many patients have a disease by geographic areas between specified periods. The incidence rate is more suitable for studies that span across different periods and for detecting changes in disease onset. Mortality and morbidity data can be aggregated by administrative boundaries to link up with census data by the Census and Statistics Bureau.

Various national and international organizations and health institutions maintain disease registers. The U.S. National Center for Health Statistics, for example, serves as the collaborating center for the World Health Organization in devising the family of International Classifications of Diseases (ICD) for North America and its use, interpretation, and periodic revision. The ICD is adopted by countries worldwide in reporting disease cases to the World Health Organization through International Health Regulations requiring routine disease notification. The ICD coupled with data from reporting countries allow for visualization and progressive tracking of global diseases. Such global cooperation not only allows a disease to gravitate to its true relative importance but also promotes transparency in global surveillance of communicable diseases.[10]

A number of questions must be considered in assembling and preparing digital data for spatial epidemiological studies using a GIS. These questions help establish the relevance or utility and reliability of the data in a study. These questions also form the basis of metadata (i.e., data about data) to provide potential users a better understanding of the data on hand.

Questions about data characteristics
- For which purpose were the data compiled?
- Are the contents relevant to the study on hand?
- What is the area coverage of the data?
- What was the density of observations used for the data compilation?

- To which map scales were the data digitized?
- Which projection, coordinate system, and datum were used?
- What is the age of the data?
- In what format are the data kept?

Questions about data quality

- How and was there data quality check?
- How accurate are positional and attribute features?
- Do the data seem logical and consistent?
- Do cartographic representations look "clean"?

Questions about data sources

- Where do data come from?
- From what medium were they originally produced?
- What is the reliability of the data provider?

2.4   Georeferencing Locational Information

Aspatial or attribute data are linked to spatial data in a GIS via a common identifier. The spatial data provide the locational information, whereas the aspatial data provide a description that may characterize the location. To be meaningful, the content descriptions must be in "natural" languages and not in encrypted codes. For example, an address location of 40.7°N and 110.3°E has little meaning to most people, whereas "27 Queens Road Central" is much clearer. At the same time, the operation of a GIS must be intuitive rather than obscure. That is to say, the sequence of computer operations should be more cognitive in nature. How then can we assign locational referencing to an event or incident in the least intimidating or awkward manner?

First, let us examine how locational referencing of an event or incident is usually done. The most direct means of assigning or obtaining a locational reference of a position is by means of a handheld GPS unit. However, each location must be surveyed or visited, and this may not be feasible in situations involving a large number of sites, as in the case of a disease outbreak or inaccessible locations in remote areas. In many situations, geocoding or address matching is a widely used method for linking a street or building address with a coordinate system for mapping (Figure 2.6). Here, each address in the patient register is furnished with an x and y coordinate pair extracted from a master address list to enable plotting of the street/building locations on a map.

Geocoding is an essential first step toward turning geographic data into useful information. Each geocoded location may represent a disease occurrence,

Patient Register

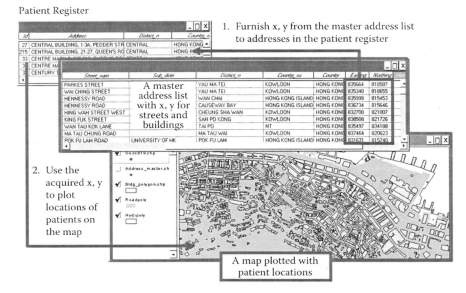

FIGURE 2.6
A color version of this figure follows page 108 Address matching or geocoding.

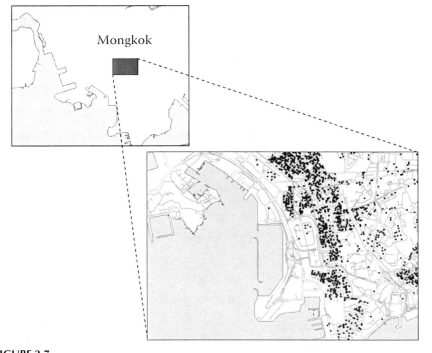

FIGURE 2.7
A point pattern distribution of patient locations. (Data from Hong Kong Lands Department and Hospital Authority.)

and the spatial arrangement of these point locations should reveal a distributional pattern (Figure 2.7). Such a map is instrumental not only in revealing disease clusters but also in the visual detection of outliers.[11,12] Additional mapping and spatial analysis techniques presented in subsequent chapters can reveal the underlying relationships, as in the example where childhood leukemia exhibited a spatial connection with nuclear power plants.[13]

2.4.1 Geocoding Problems

Geocoding is traditionally achieved by using network or street addresses.[14] In many countries where street networks are not available or do not comply with the U.S. TIGER data structure[15] as in the case of Hong Kong, it may be easier to compile a comprehensive and georeferenced address database (the master list with point coordinates) based either on building or street names. Geocoding can then be realized by using the master list against which an address entry is compared and matched (see Figure 2.6). In this case, address entries in a patient register are required to conform to some data input standard. Our experience with the Hong Kong data has uncovered a number of geocoding problems resulting from inconsistencies in address entries (Table 2.3). Such inconsistencies became a major obstacle in automated address matching and resulted in only about 30% correct match on first run. The match rate was increased by another 35% after careful editing of address entries by local experts. The remaining 35% of addresses required intense human labor to be locatable on maps, with about 3% remaining unknown or invalid.

We discovered that more than 30% of the addresses in the database were spelled erroneously, leading to locational misspecification. These errors were largely attributed to the lack of quality control at the input stage where, in most cases, hospital receptionists who keyed in the data did not know the proper names of selected residential buildings and resorted to using the phonetic equivalents. Although both online and printed telephone directories and street maps were available for cross-referencing, there was no established policy requiring the verification of patient addresses. Furthermore, some unintentional mistakes in spelling were also present.

Of particular note is that a third of the errors in address encoding arose out of differences in the nonstandardized naming protocols of buildings. Edifices in Hong Kong are labeled as houses, mansions, estates, courts, villages, or villas. There is no clear definition of these labels, and the naming of buildings seems to hinge on the preference of property developers. This inherent inconsistency seems to cause a great deal of confusion in address matching as illustrated in Table 2.3. A further complication comes from nonunique building names: some buildings located in different districts use the same name. These problems could be easily resolved if district name were to become a mandatory field in the data entry process. We provide several recommendations for address standardization:

TABLE 2.3

Problems in Address Entries

Types of Errors	Incorrect	Correct
I. Homonyms	Chung **Yiu** Hse	Chung **Yew** Hse
	Fuk Hoi Hse	**Fook** Hoi Hse
	Fanling Lau	**Fan Leng** Lau
	Hoi **Koon** Mansion	Hoi **Kwun** Mansion
	Shan Shui Hse	**San** Shui Hse
	Wah **Tsui** Hse	Wah **Chui** Hse
	Yiu **Shun** Hse	Yiu **Chun** Hse
II. Phonetic translation	**Fung Yu Bldg**	**Harvest Mansion**
	Kam Fai Crt	**Golden Glory**
	Hoi Yan Gdn	Grand Horizon
	Ng Chau Bldg	**Continental Mansion**
	Tai Wo Gdn	**Treasure** Gdn
	Pik Lai Crt	Believe Gdn
	Wang On Crt	**Winner Hse**
III. Carelessness or input errors	123 Tai **Nam** St	123 Tai **Nan** St
	25e **Polar** St	25e **Poplar** St
	38 Kennedy Town **Traya**	38 Kennedy Town **Praya**
	Laguan City	**Laguna** City
	Saddie Ridge Gdn	**Saddle** Ridge Gdn
	Tin **Ling** Hse	Tin **Ning** Hse
IV. Naming system		
1. Building	Chung Mei **Hse**	Chung Mei **Bldg**
	Yuet Ming **Hse**	Yuet Ming **Bldg**
2. Sun Chuen	Fung Wong **Est**	Fung Wong **Sun Chuen**
	Lok Man **Est**	Lok Man **Sun Chuen**
3. Court	Ho Ming **Yuen**	Ho Ming **Crt**
	Yen Po **Hse**	Yen Po **Crt**
	Reve **Crt**	Reve **Plaza**
4. Lau	Kam Shan **Hse**	Kam Shan **Lau**
	Kwun Lung **Hse**	Kwun Lung **Lau**
5. Mansion	Cheung Fai **Bldg**	Cheung Fai **Mansion**
	Yick Lee **Bldg**	Yick Lee **Mansion**
6. Village	43 Tin Sum **Tsuen**	43 Tin Sam **Village**
	Ling Shan **Vill**	Ling Shan **Tsuen**
7. Others	22 Yuk Wah **Crescent**	22 Yuk Wah **Lane**
	City One **Hse**	City One **Plaza**

Force all entries into capital letters.

Abolish commas or symbols separating the words.

Omit flat and floor numbers.

Adopt standardized abbreviations wherever possible.

Consider the first occurrences of road number.

Consider suffixes (e.g., A, B, East, West) as a separate item.

2.4.2   Choosing the Right Address

In spatial epidemiological studies, the choice of a suitable address (whether residential, place of employment, school, or recreational) may affect the representativeness of a disease pattern. The current practice of using residential addresses tends to overstate the effects of the home environment and understate those of the work or school environment in disease accounting because many individuals may spend more time at work and children may spend more time at school than at home. This customary practice arises out of convenience because patient records contain only residential addresses. Given the growing improvements in technology, it seems likely that other nodalities where people spend their time could be incorporated into a more robust disease tracking system in the future.

Geocoding is imperative to the mapping and analysis of disease records. Local health organizations must first standardize the process of data capture, especially of address entries, whereas cost-effective procedures and protocols for handling and managing data update also must be established. The need for a constant and sustained investment in health informatics will ensure continued and more standardized development of spatial epidemiological mapping and analysis.

2.5   Aggregating Geographic Data

Although it is possible to obtain point-based data representing disease occurrences as indicated in Sections 2.3 and 2.4, a point distribution map such as that in Figure 2.7 is difficult to interpret and often not a desirable option for policy makers. Moreover, such detailed data are not suitable for public release, given concerns over personal privacy and data confidentiality. Units of aggregation typically used by many public health agencies are census enumeration units. These not only provide an acceptable solution to ensure the protection of data privacy and the individual's anonymity but also allow for the incorporation of demographic and socioeconomic analysis of the enumeration units within which disease events take place.

2.5.1   Units of Aggregation

The use of census enumeration units for analysis is common among early studies in spatial epidemiology. Census data provide a basis for understanding the demographic constructs and socioeconomic characteristics of the study population. Although a detailed discussion of the census is beyond the scope of this book, the census geography of Hong Kong is worth mentioning because of the examples used in the following chapters. Census enumeration units adopted by different countries may differ. For example, province/state, county, and townships are the units used in North American and many European nations, but these configurations are not suitable for regions of small areal coverage such as Hong Kong and Macau.

In Hong Kong, the enumeration units for the population census are arranged in three hierarchical levels, from the least to the most detailed: Secondary Planning Units (SPUs), Tertiary Planning Units (TPUs), and Street Block Planning Units (SBUs). The boundaries of TPUs and SBUs are, for the most part, recognizable across the Hong Kong landscape through the formation of water bodies, streets, railways, and other man-made or natural features. Other than the three spatial hierarchies, census data can also be reconstituted into DC districts and their constituency areas (DCCA). In the 2001 census year, Hong Kong was divided into 18 DCs, 9 SPUs, 282 TPUs, and 2,627 SBUs. Similar to other nations, there are additional enumeration units created for different purposes, for example, electoral or school board districts.

Figure 2.8 shows SBU zoning in the Mongkok area of Hong Kong. The zoning of SBUs more or less follows major road arteries such as Nathan Road and Mongkok Road. Such a zoning method is convenient for temporal analysis because roads in an established district rarely change. The figure also shows that SBUs are essentially small and measure about 0.024 km^2 in size — except for units 229/01 and 229/52, which are the results of the rapid reclamation work along the shoreline of Tai Kok Tsui.

The case of Thailand is similar to many countries. The census enumeration units of Thailand are arranged hierarchically into 76 changwat (province), 926 amphoe (district), and 7,410 tumbon (subdistrict).

2.5.2   Data Aggregation Concerns

Point representation is used to portray health data at the most detailed level of geographic space. In spatial epidemiological studies, the plotting of disease locations as points may reveal its distributional pattern, but points, in and of themselves, are not sufficient to disclose the possible causes or interactions with other factors. Further analyses incorporating sociodemographic and environmental factors are usually desirable. These analyses can require disease counts by locations to be aggregated to some census enumeration units (e.g., province or state, county, township, village) where summary statistics on the socioeconomic composition of these units (e.g., age and gender

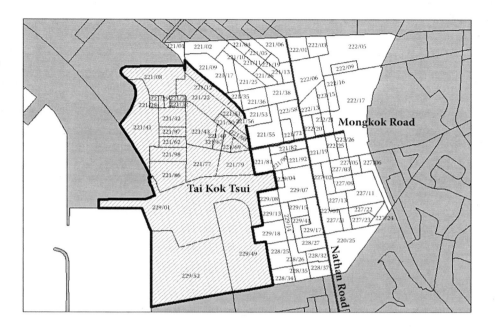

FIGURE 2.8
A sample of street block units in Mongkok, Hong Kong. (Data from Hong Kong Lands Department.)

groups, median income, educational attainment) can be studied to supplement the analyses (Figure 2.9). Other statistical adjustments to help refine point data analysis, such as kernel density estimation and smoothing, are discussed in other chapters.

Census data that characterize geographic areas often offer an important resource to further examine possible associations between the living environment and health outcomes. For example, Xie et al.[16] found that high levels of parental education and family income in seven cities over four regions (including Harbin and Shenyang in the northeast, Wuhan in the central region, Chengdu and Kungming in the southwest, and Hangzhou and Qingdao in the coastal areas) were significant risk factors for overweight prevalence in Chinese adolescents. However, the results could vary depending on how the areal units are configured and often referred to as the MAUP (Figure 2.10).[17–19]

The aggregation of point data into areal data "ignores" a large amount of locational information in the observed point distribution. This aggregation may inadvertently mask true hot spots as high frequencies, such as those along shared borders, thus distributing clusters among adjacent areas. The process may also result in a more "uniform" or smoothed areal distribution of events across space than would have been observed through point pat-

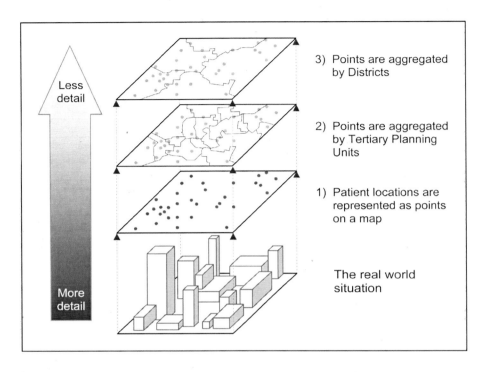

FIGURE 2.9
Aggregation of epidemiological observations for mapping.

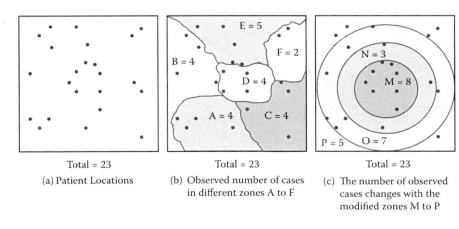

FIGURE 2.10
The modifiable areal unit problem.

terns, as in Figure 2.10 where zones A to E register rather similar numbers of observed cases.

In practice, we must exercise caution when interpreting the results of area-based statistics because of problems arising from variable scales, different enumeration units or boundaries, ecological fallacy, and the MAUP.[17] Aggregated data may overestimate or underestimate a phenomenon, especially for marginal cases in the vicinity of defined boundaries. This circumstance might also give rise to double counting or omission of some incidents in computerized and GIS processing when formulating statistical indicators across a selected time frame.

2.6 Summary

GIS applications typically rely on data from multiple sources, and they are very data-intensive. Because GIS data development can be costly, it is essential to establish partnership to share or access data from external sources where available. In many cases, sociodemographic and environmental data can be obtained or purchased, but data about disease or health care services may not be readily available or easily accessible. The use of sensitive data in epidemiological studies also necessitates data aggregation, an additional step for protecting data confidentiality.

It is perhaps appropriate to end this chapter with the statement made by Professor David Rhind as food for thought.

> GIS is not simply the geographical equivalent of word processing. It is a way of integrating information from different sources and doing so in a way which is underpinned by good science. From this comes added value: the range of questions which can be addressed expands very rapidly as the number of data sets safely linked together is increased.

> **David Rhind, CBE**
> *Vice Chancellor of City University, London*

References

1. Burrough, P.A., and McDonnell, R.A., *Principles of Geographical Information Systems*, Oxford University Press, Oxford, 1998.
2. Snyder, J.P., *Flattening the Earth — Two Thousand Years of Map Projections*, University of Chicago Press, Chicago, IL, 1993.

3. Mark, D., and Egenhofer, M., Modeling spatial relations between lines and regions: combining formal mathematical models and human subjects testing, *Cartography and Geographical Information Systems*, 21, 195, 1994.

4. Jensen, J.R., *Introductory Digital Image Processing*, 3rd ed., Prentice Hall, Upper Saddle River, NJ, 2005.

5. Elliott, P., Wakefield, J., Best, N., and Briggs, D., Eds., *Spatial Epidemiology: Methods and Applications*, Oxford University Press, Oxford, 2000.

6. So, F.M., *An Application of Geographic Information Systems in the Study of Spatial Epidemiology of Respiratory Diseases in Hong Kong, 1996–2000*, M.Phil. thesis, University of Hong Kong, Hong Kong, 2002.

7. Bowling, A., *Research Methods in Health: Investigating Health and Health Services*, Open University Press, Philadelphia, PA, 1997.

8. Meade, M.S., and Earickson, R.J., *Medical Geography*, Guildford Press, London, 2000.

9. Waller, L.A., and Gotway, C.A., *Applied Spatial Statistics for Public Health Data*, Wiley, Hoboken, NJ, 2004.

10. Obijiofor, A., International law and communicable diseases, *Bulletin of the World Health Organization*, 80(12), 946, 2002.

11. Bailey, T.C., and Gatrell, A.C., *Interactive Spatial Data Analysis*, Longman, Harlow, 1995.

12. Diggle, P., *Statistical Analysis of Spatial Point Patterns*, Arnold, London, 2003.

13. Openshaw, S., Craft, A.E., Charlton, M., and Birch, J.M., Preliminary communication: investigation of leukemia clusters by the use of a geographical analysis machine, *Lancet*, 1, 272, 1988.

14. Rushton, G., and Armstrong, M.P., *Improving Public Health Through Geographical Information Systems: An Instructional Guide to Major Concepts and Their Implementation*, 1997, Web Version 1.0. Available: http://www.uiowa.edu/~geog/health/index7.html [accessed on June 4, 2007].

15. U.S. Census Bureau, *TIGER/Line Files Technical Documentation*, 2003. Available: http://www.census.gov/geo/www/tiger/tgrcd108/tgr108cd.pdf [accessed on June 4, 2007].

16. Xie, B., Chou, C.P., Spruijt-Metz, D., Reynolds, K., Palmer, P.H., Gallaher, P., Clark, P., Sun, P., Guo, Q., and Johnson, C.A., Socio-demographic and economic correlates of overweight status in Chinese adolescents, *American Journal of Health Behavior*, 31(4), 339, 2007.

17. Openshaw, S., *The Modifiable Areal Unit Problem*, Geobooks, Norwich, CT, 1984.

18. Rushton, G., Improving the geographical basis of health surveillance using GIS, in *GIS and Health*, Gatrell, A.G., and Loytonen, M., Eds., Taylor & Francis, London, 1998, Chap. 5.

19. Gatrell, A.C., *Geographies of Health: An Introduction*, Blackwell, Oxford, 2002.

3

Spatial Analysis Software and Methods

3.1 Introduction

The discipline of geography contributes to the study of spatial epidemiology through the description and understanding of the spatial variations of disease risks.[1] Disease mapping is the first step in undertaking descriptive spatial analysis. Supplementing descriptive analysis with geospatial and geostatistical methods allows for further examination of spatial variations in possible risk factors leading to disease outcomes. This chapter provides an overview of the GIS software, data set, and spatial analysis methods often used for health-related analyses.

3.2 Software

There is a wide selection of GIS software available for visualizing, analyzing, creating, and managing spatial data that offer single-user desktop, server network, or Web solutions. They have also appropriate open-application programming interfaces and support key data interchange formats and Web service standards for ensuring relevant GIS and IT interoperability between systems over wired and/or wireless networks. Major market players (in alphabetical order) include such names as ArcGIS, AutoCAD, Geomedia, MapInfo, MicroStation, Microsoft Mapping, and Oracle Spatial. These software provide comprehensive GIS analytical functionality features and are licensed commercially.

Some GIS-like software with limited analytical functions have been customized to suit the basic geographic needs of health professionals. For instance, Epi Info and Epi Map are public domain mapping software designed for the global community of public health practitioners and researchers. Both provide a simplistic approach for database construction, data entry, and analysis with results shown as epidemiological statistics, maps, and graphs. Although Epi Info is a trademark of the U.S. Centers for Disease Control and

Prevention (CDC), the programs, documentation, and teaching materials are in the public domain for free distribution in different languages.

To assist readers in carrying out health analyses covered in this book, we have adopted GIS freeware in all examples. Specifically, we use CrimeStat, GeoDa, and HealthMapper in our demonstrations. The characteristic features of these freeware are described in the sections that follow.

3.2.1 CrimeStat

CrimeStat is a spatial statistics program for the analysis of crime incident locations.[2] The program was developed by Ned Levine and Associates and funded by grants from the National Institute of Justice. CrimeStat is Windows-based, and it interfaces with most desktop GIS programs. It comprises tools for point data mapping and spatial analytical functions, including cluster analysis tools to locate hot spots. Its purpose is to provide supplemental statistical tools to aid law enforcement agencies and criminal justice researchers in their crime mapping and strategic planning efforts. Because it is more of a spatial statistical software than a mapping program, some of the textual and tabular outputs of CrimeStat must be imported into software such as GeoDa or HealthMapper (discussed below) for visual displays.

CrimeStat is used by many police departments in the United States as well as by criminal justice and other researchers worldwide. The executable version of CrimeStat III (Version 3.1) is downloadable from http://www.icpsr. umich.edu/CRIMESTAT/download.htm. Its installation is menu-driven and straightforward upon acceptance of the user agreement (Figure 3.1).

3.2.2 GeoDa

GeoDa is an interactive environment that combines maps with statistical charts and graphics, using the technology of dynamically linked windows.[3] It was developed by Luc Anselin of the Spatial Analysis Laboratory of the University of Illinois, Urbana–Champaign. Along with its mapping functionality, GeoDa contains the usual EDA graphs (i.e., EDA graphics including histogram, box plot, scatterplot, etc.) and implements brushing for both maps and statistical plots. Maps can be constructed from points as well as polygons, and tools are provided to create one from another (e.g., centroid computation from polygons, Thiessen polygons from points) as well as to set up various types of spatial weights for the analytical models.

GeoDa is used extensively for teaching spatial analytical methods and has proven itself useful in undergraduate education by providing instructors access to a free tool for exploratory data analysis in the classroom. The beta release is free for download for noncommercial use only from http://www. geoda.uiuc.edu/. You can subscribe to the Open Space mailing list to find out about bug fixes and new releases. Once downloaded, the installation procedure of GeoDa practically runs by itself (Figure 3.2).

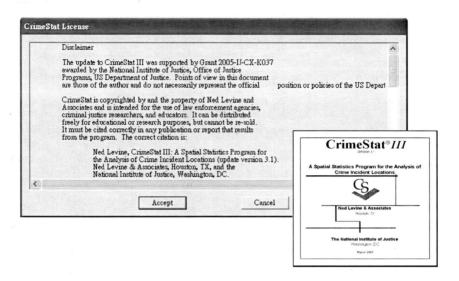

FIGURE 3.1
Accessing and installing CrimeStat.

3.2.3 HealthMapper

The HealthMapper is a surveillance and mapping application, developed by the World Health Organization (WHO), which aims at addressing critical surveillance information needs across infectious disease programs at the national and global levels. It has a user-friendly data management and mapping system customized specifically for public health users. The system not only facilitates data standardization and the collection and updating of epidemiological data but also emphasizes interventions while providing immediate visualization of surveillance data in the form of maps, tables, and charts. In 2003, the system began to support the surveillance of HIV/AIDS/STI and tuberculosis, control of communicable diseases in complex emergency situations, outbreak alert and response, and an integrated management of childhood illnesses. The system is currently in operation to support a range of infectious diseases in more than 60 countries in all regions of the WHO.[4]

HealthMapper can be obtained through written application to the WHO (Public Health Mapping and GIS Team, 1211 Geneva 27, Switzerland, or via e-mail to health_mapping@who.int) with details of your organization and how the requested data will be used. The program comes in two CDs with a packaged database of countries of interest to the user, including core baseline geographic, demographic, and health information covering the location of communities and health care and education facilities, accessibility by roads, access to safe water, and population demography. Software installation is menu-driven and straightforward (Figure 3.3).

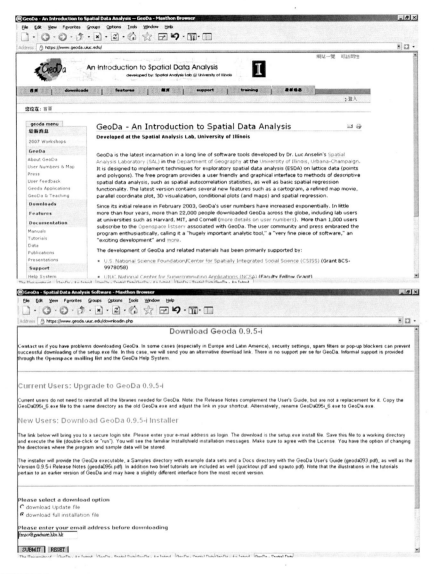

FIGURE 3.2
Accessing and installing GeoDa.

3.2.4 Summary

The freeware listed above are designed for specific purposes and do not contain a full set of functions normally available in commercial software. As can be seen from our examples in Chapters 4 to 6, it is sometimes necessary to conduct spatial analytical procedures in one software (e.g., using CrimeStat to undertake cluster analysis or compute standard deviational ellipses

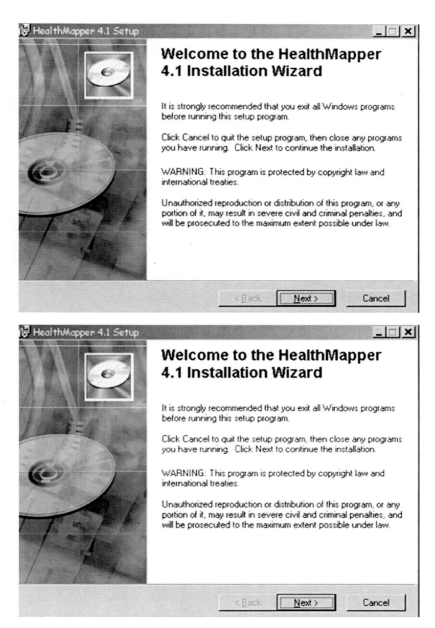

FIGURE 3.3
Installing HealthMapper.

(SDEs) and use another program (e.g., GeoDa or HealthMapper) to display the results. Readily available to users, these freeware complement and supplement each other in spatial analytical methods and data visualization.

3.3 Data Sets

Our examples throughout this book make use of data from two geographic areas: Hong Kong and Thailand (see also Chapter 2, Section 2.1). In the case of Hong Kong, we study hospital admission records for 1996–2000 obtained from 44 public hospitals under the management of the Hong Kong Hospital Authority. The admission records contain four categories of patient details: personal (SEX and DOB), address (BLDG at the building level), disease code (ICD), and dates of admission (DOA) and discharge (DOD). We selected records of patients admitted for asthma using ICD code 493. A total of 12,853 unique cases were extracted, after we eliminated 754 cases of repeated admissions of the same patients. Table B.1 in Appendix B summarizes the items and values of the asthma cases. They are stored in DBF format for further processing in Chapter 5. These cases offer an extremely good representation of asthma cases in Hong Kong because 90% of its population sought health care from public hospitals. The remaining 10% of the population, largely composed of well-to-do families, chose private health care.

We also compiled from newspaper sources cases of severe acute respiratory syndrome (SARS) reported between April 1 and May 15, 2003. These represented official episodes confirmed by the Hong Kong Department of Health on a daily basis (CDATE) for the said period. The data were recorded at the building level (B_NAME, BLOCK, and STREET) but did not contain personal details of the infected individuals as did the asthma cases. The relevant attributes are listed in Table B.2 in Appendix B.

In the case of Thailand, we use the 2004 dengue data provided by the Thailand Ministry of Public Health (Table B.3 in Appendix B). Although the data contain personal details about individual patients (SEX, AGE, RACE, and OCCU), they come without specific addresses, thus rendering point-based analysis infeasible. The data, however, can be summarized into area-based statistics according to different administrative units.

In addition, the feature type, data structure, and sources of extra data for the two study areas are as listed in Tables B.4, B.5, and B.6 in Appendix B. These data are needed for map presentation, visualization, and other purposes. For instance, the pollution monitoring sites established by the Environmental Protection Department of the government of Hong Kong SAR are of the point feature type, and their accompanying air pollution records are needed for examining relationships between air quality and respiratory illnesses. Both the 1996 Tertiary Planning Unit (TPU) and District Council (DC) boundaries from the Lands Department of the Hong Kong SAR government are of the polygon feature type, and they are needed to support the overlay operation and aggregate point data for areal-based analysis. In the case of Thailand, administrative boundaries come in four levels: changwat (province), amphoe (district), tumbon (subdistrict), and village.

TABLE 3.1

A Summary of Data Description and Their Sources

Data	Source	Feature Type	Data Format	Table in Appendix
Hong Kong				
Hospital admission records, 1996–2000	Hong Kong Hospital Authority	Attribute	XLS	B.1
SARS	Various newspapers	Point	SHP	B.2
Pollution monitoring sites	Environmental Protection Department, HKSAR	Point	SHP	B.4
Tertiary planning unit	Census and Statistics Department, HKSAR, and Survey and Mapping Office, Lands Department, HKSAR	Polygon	SHP	B.5
DC				B.6
Demographic		Attribute	XLS	—
Socioeconomic				
Thailand				
Dengue disease	Bureau of Epidemiology of Thailand	Point	XLS	B.3
Village	Royal Thai Survey Department via Bureau of Epidemiology of Thailand	Polygon	SHP	B.7
Tumbon				B.8
Amphoe				B.9
Changwat				B.10

Table 3.1 summarizes the different input data used in our illustrations in Chapters 4 to 6. The data are of varied scales and reliability, which reflect the true situation in practice. In some cases, as in the preparation of the SARS data, considerable preprocessing was needed to undertake data conversion and aggregation before data were rendered useful. These essential steps are not described in the book.

3.4 Spatial Analysis

What distinguishes a GIS from other information systems is its collection of spatial analytical functions.[5] The steps involve, first, the formulation of a study question and the identification of a study area. Next comes the need to identify sources of spatial and disease data for inclusion in a GIS. The procedures to manipulate and process the data depend very much on the purpose of the study and the functionalities of the selected GIS software.

The sequence of operational procedures for GIS-based health-related analyses is outlined below.

Step 1: What is my study question? Example: "Is there a correlation between asthma and low income?"

Step 2: Where is my study area? Example: Territory of Hong Kong.

Step 3: Which spatial data do I need to collect and what are the available data formats? Example: Administrative boundaries of Hong Kong by DC districts or TPUs, buildings, roads, coastlines, and so forth. Refer to Table 2.1 for a list of spatial data formats.

What are some possible data sources? Example: Government agencies (such as those listed in Table 3.1) or private companies. If there is more than one data source, are the data using the same projection or coordinate system and for the same map scale?

Are the spatial data ready to use? Do I need to amend or add to them? Example: Data conversion to conform to a selected format, georeferencing an image, and adding or removing features from digital spatial data.

Step 4: Which type of disease or additional data do I need to collect? Example: Hospital admission records, clinical, and survey or census data.

What measurement items do I need? Example: Disease counts, date of discharge, disease codes, and so forth.

Do I have addresses to link disease records to spatial data? Example: Incidence or surrogate locations (represented by residential, work, play, or school addresses).

Do I need to undertake data computation or standardization? Example: Population density, age–sex adjustment, and mortality or morbidity measures.

Step 5: Which software should I use or acquire given specific requirements? Appendix A offers a list of software choices.

Do I need to perform geocoding or address matching? Example: Address matching at which geographic level(s), whether by point, building, street block, or district?

Do I need to do geostatistical or time-series analyses? Example: Compute and plot mean centers of disease clusters or create streaming videos.

Step 6: Which types of spatial analyses are appropriate? Example: area aggregation, geographic queries, neighborhood analyses, spatial overlay, spatial autocorrelation, spatiotemporal changes, and geostatistical analysis.

At which geographic level(s) will I present my results? Example: *point*-based or aggregated by districts or other spatial units.

In reference to Step 6 above, three types of spatial analysis are suitable for examining epidemiological data: (1) disease mapping of points and areas, (2) spatial autocorrelation, and (3) geostatistical analysis. They are arranged in increasing levels of operational complexity. The first process involves an exploratory and elementary analysis to estimate regional disease risks and detect areal biases. The second process of spatial autocorrelation attempts to assess the level of interdependence between a variable and its spatial location. The third process strives to provide accurate and reliable estimations of a natural incident at locations where no measurement is available. However, before arriving at Step 6, there is usually a need to undertake data standardization in Step 4, whereby the same population distribution is applied to each geographic area being compared.

3.4.1   Age–Sex Standardization

The simplest method for calculating the ratio of a disease in an area within a specified period is by using the crude rate. The crude death rate, for example, is defined as the total number of deaths for all ages divided by the population. However, crude rates can be misleading because of differential population characteristics, especially the age–sex difference. The crude death rate of a geographic area may be high simply because of a higher proportion of elderly people living in the area. There is also the need to standardize by gender, given that males are known to have a shorter life expectancy than females.[6]

Two common methods for age–sex adjustment known as the direct and indirect methods were introduced in the nineteenth century.[6,7] The direct method is preferred because it preserves consistency between populations and is deemed appropriate for comparing groups or examining trends across multiple periods using the same standard population. Widespread use of the direct method was observed in the United States, especially by the National Cancer Institute in studying the geographic distribution of various cancers.[8] However, the selection of an appropriate standard population is to some extent arbitrary because no "correct" standard population exists,[9] and this method cannot be used if the study population is unknown or unavailable. In the United States, most current government statistics standardize on the year 2000 population.

Indirect standardization and its corresponding indices, such as the Standardized Mortality Ratio (SMR), were only used 30 years after the introduction of the direct method (1853). The formula for computing SMR follows:

$$\text{SMR} = \frac{N}{\sum R_{si} P_i} \qquad [3.1]$$

where

N = total number of patients in the observed population

R_{si} = age–gender specific mortality rate in age–gender interval i in the standard population

P_i = the population of age–gender interval i in the observed population.

The indirect method of standardization requires only the population at risk in each age group and the total number of deaths in the study population, which makes it a convenient substitute for the deficient direct method. Furthermore, this method has the advantage of a lower standard error as explained by Inskip et al.[8] The SMR is the first approximation to this estimate, and this index is useful when there are small numbers of events in the study population leading to unstable death rates and large errors of estimation. The indirect method of rate standardization appears to offer advantages for small area planning and resource allocation.

3.4.2 Disease Mapping

Tobler's first law of geography, which states that "things that are closer are more related," is central to core spatial analytical techniques as well as analytical conceptions of geographic space.[10] In the case of disease spread, individuals near or exposed to a contagious person or a tainted environmental setting are deemed more susceptible to certain types of illnesses.[11,12] Cartographic design and mapping techniques can draw attention to these locations by displaying an aggregation or lack of such events or patterns in space. Cartographic presentation and design has the following framework: (1) geographic feature classification, (2) scale determination, (3) symbol categorization, and (4) graphic primitives (Figure 3.4). The basic working units of disease data include point (e.g., patient locations), line (e.g., transmission route), and area (e.g., disease rate by county). Depending on the data scaling

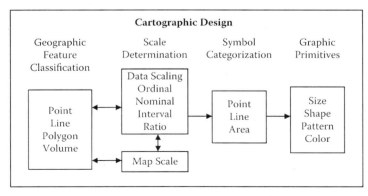

FIGURE 3.4
A framework of cartographic design. (Adapted from Muehrcke and Muehrcke,[13] and Campbell.[14])

and level of measurement (whether nominal, ordinal, interval, or ratio), the use of certain combinations of symbols and graphic primitives is more effective in conveying spatial distributions.[13,14]

In spatial epidemiology, point-based data representing disease or patient locations are the bases of data collection. Geocoded point data derived from address matching (as discussed in Section 2.4 of Chapter 2) form the essential input for disease mapping. Very often, disease mapping involves making maps of point and choropleth patterns (Figure 3.5). Although it is appropriate in secure research settings to represent locations of disease incidence at the local scale, for example, to search for possible disease clusters, point maps for public distribution and consumption may be deemed too revealing and sensitive.

Health events for small geographic areas are recorded in traditional approaches as preset areal units.[15] Although point pattern representation is a quasi-accurate account of a health event, its use is undesirable in portraying disease occurrences of acute sensitivity (such as AIDS and SARS). To safeguard personal privacy and curtail social segregation, point-based data are collapsed by enumeration units for visual presentation (as in choropleth, proportional symbol, and cartogram methods). Aggregating point data by a set of areal units allows distributional maps to be created to reveal new insights.[16] The point-in-polygon operation in a GIS, for example, can aggregate point data by administrative zones. However, the selection of which boundary files to overlay with the point data must be done with care to reduce misspecification of case with at-risk populations (see also Section 2.5 of Chapter 2).[17]

Identification and discrimination between map symbols are necessary to represent data in a meaningful way. Clear and intuitive map symbols are the main components to allow map viewers a visual understanding of the resultant pattern or intended message. A variety of thematic mapping or visualization techniques are available, and they have been discussed thoroughly.[18,19] Other than point pattern maps, the most commonly used mapping technique is by means of choropleth or shaded area mapping (Figure 3.5). This method involves grouping numerical values (e.g., disease rate per 1,000, standard deviation) associated with some enumeration units (e.g., census tracts) into ordinal classes (e.g., five ranked classes representing very high, high, medium, low, and very low readings). Each group is assigned a color in which the darker color represents a higher value and lighter color a lower value. Each enumeration area is shaded the color of its corresponding class containing the value. To reduce adverse visualization effects projected by small areas of high values or large areas of small values, it is recommended that this technique be used to map rates instead of raw readings.

Variations of the choropleth method include the proportional symbol or chart maps and the area cartograms (Figure 3.5). The proportional symbol method displays rate data using geometric shapes (circles, squares, or bar charts) sized according to the values or classes being represented. Likewise, the area cartogram stretches or shrinks an enumeration area according to

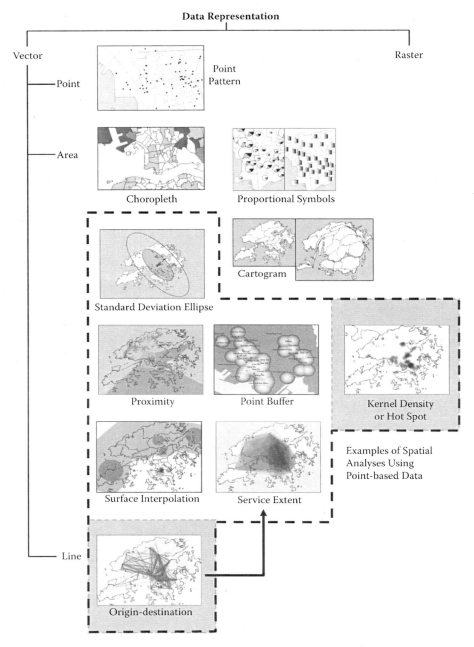

FIGURE 3.5
Types of spatial analytical map outputs.

its value to highlight numerical differences among the regions. The greater difference there is between the values under representation and the absolute size of an enumeration area (e.g., a large value over a small area or vice versa), the more deformation is evident between the resultant and original maps. Hence, area cartograms are often presented alongside an undistorted original shape to render proper interpretation.

The remaining mapping techniques illustrated in Figure 3.5 are used to portray results of spatial analytical functions. The examples show a variation of mapping techniques arising from point-based data. They offer uniquely different visualization of disease or health-related patterns, development, and trends. For example, the kernel density method is a means of summarizing points by quadrants or grids of a uniform size (instead of some administrative zones) through a moving window approach. This method of presentation not only addresses the issue of data privacy but also diminishes the effects of MAUP and area dependence. Point buffers may also be used to indicate more clearly the patterns of spatial clustering of points and delineate possible hot spot areas. The choice of suitable mapping techniques relies largely on cartographic experience and geographic understanding, in addition to creativity on the part of the spatial analyst.

Disease mapping is the first step toward understanding the spatial aspects of health-related problems because particular types of information are highlighted in maps.[20,21] Disease distributions can be shown through different cartographic symbolization as points, lines, and patterns. Associative analyses can then be formulated through visual inspection of the disease maps in conjunction with statistical deduction. Howe[22] stressed that the intention of disease mapping was to display the answer to the question "where?" but not "why there?" Although disease mapping seems only a tool for preliminary data exploration, it nonetheless offers useful hints in terms of informing needs for further statistical and empirical analyses as well as different visualization techniques.

In general, areal mapping filters or masks individual information through data aggregation and has been widely used for data released in the public domain. However, we must recognize that point data are the foundation for many spatial analytical approaches, as depicted in Figure 3.5. Various spatial analyses and their corresponding visualization techniques offer significant exploratory power in probing a health situation and its development. We shall illustrate how these techniques are applicable in epidemiological studies in ensuing chapters.

3.4.3 Spatial Autocorrelation

The hypotheses about the etiology of a disease can be formulated, and risk factors can also be examined by taking into account the spatial variation of diseases. It has been demonstrated that geography could offer much to the medical knowledge through what is generally termed *associative occurrences*.[23] Statistical explanation and disease maps form the methodological framework to understand associative occurrences between possible disease covariates and the disease. The statistical explanation ranges from a simple χ^2 test of significance to complex multivariate explanations. In epidemiology, a disease may be modeled with specific mathematical approaches and quantification. The formulated hypotheses can then be statistically tested by rigorous methods, such as intervention, cohort, and case-control studies.

One of the major sources for generating hypotheses of etiology is through the use of disease maps. The method of spatial autocorrelation is essentially an operation involving an assessment of interdependence between two variables, that is, a variable in reference to its spatial location.[3] Spatial autocorrelation methods look for the presence of systematic pattern in the spatial distribution of a variable (Figure 3.6). If nearby or neighboring areas are more alike, there is positive spatial autocorrelation. Negative spatial autocorrelation describes patterns in which neighboring areas are unlike. Spatial autocorrelation can be measured in terms of indices such as Moran's I and Geary's C, also illustrated in Figure 3.6. These measures will be discussed further in Chapter 5.

3.4.4   Geostatistical Analysis

Back in the mid-1960s, geostatistics was applied primarily to problems in geology and mining. Today, geostatistics provides a methodology for interpolating data of an irregular pattern but also can be understood as an "application of probabilistic methods to regionalized variables."[24] Geostatistics concerns issues of spatial contiguity whereby locations of missing values are assigned estimated values from known values based on statistical accuracy and reliability. In other words, a general assumption in geostatistics is that there exist implicit links between locations and their respective data values, termed *spatial autocorrelation*.

Geostatistics has been widely adopted in environmental impact assessment, marine studies, and hydrogeology, but its application in spatial epi-

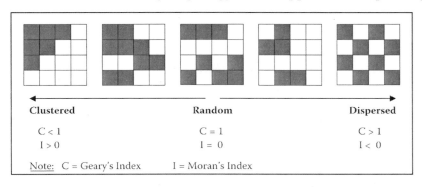

FIGURE 3.6
Spatial association and correlation.

demiology is evolving. Geostatistical methods have been used to construct maps of spatial variation in disease prevalence where health registries are not available or where survey data representative of areas are available.[25] It is a powerful tool because of its capability to characterize a spatial structure via a consistent probabilistic model or statistical smoothing algorithms. As such, the predictions made are tailored to the intrinsic structure of the spatial variable.

Geostatistics involves a set of statistical tools (histograms, trend analysis, semivariogram cloud, etc.) and, importantly, a measure of statistical reliability or uncertainty to allow a deeper understanding of the properties of data distributed in space and time to best model the data by different interpolation techniques (inverse distance weighted, spline, kriging, etc.). These tools allow an exploration of the distribution of data, global and local outliers, global trends, as well as spatial autocorrelation or directional variation. One of the most used interpolation techniques is the kriging method with the assumption of autocorrelation between sample points.

3.5 Summary

This chapter not only accounts for the software and data used in Chapters 4 to 6 of this book but also the accompanying methodologies for spatial analyses. We have introduced in this chapter three freeware for disease mapping and spatial analysis: CrimeStat, GeoDa, and HealthMapper. The disease data used in subsequent chapters are also described: (1) the 1996–2000 asthma cases from the Hong Kong Hospital Authority, (2) a sample of 2003 SARS episodes as extracted from local newspapers, and (3) the 2004 dengue disease cases of Thailand. We have also presented key procedures to undertake a GIS analysis in health studies. In the next chapter, we will visualize the point pattern distribution of our sample data on SARS and examine if the disease exhibits patterns of spatial clustering. The point-based data will be aggregated for areal-based analyses in Chapters 5 and 6.

References

1. Elliot, P., Wakefield, J.C., Best, N.G., and Briggs, D.J., *Spatial Epidemiology: Methods and Applications*, Oxford University Press, Oxford, 2000.
2. Levine, N., *CrimeStat 1.1, A Spatial Statistics Program for the Analysis of Crime Incident Locations*, National Institute of Justice, Washington, DC, 2000.

3. Anselin, L., Syabri, I., and Kho, Y., *GeoDa: An Introduction to Spatial Data Analysis*, 2004. Available: http://www.geoda.uiuc.edu/pdf/geodaGA.pdf [accessed on June 6, 2006].

4. World Health Organization, *Tools for Public Health Mapping and GIS*, 2007. Available: http://www.who.int/health_mapping/tools/healthmapper/en/ [accessed on September 9, 2007].

5. Longley, P.A., Goodchild, M.F., Maguire, D.J., and Rhind, D.W., *Geographic Information Systems and Science*, Wiley, New York, NY, 2001.

6. Bowling, A., *Research Methods in Health: Investigating Health and Health Services*, Open University Press, Philadelphia, PA, 1997.

7. Curtin, L.R., and Kelin, R.J., Direct standardisation (age-adjusted death rates), *Healthy People 2000: Statistical Notes 6*, U.S. Government Printing Office, Washington, DC, 1995.

8. Inskip, H., Beral, V., Fraser, P., and Haskey, J., Methods for age-adjustment of rates, *Statistics in Medicine*, 2, 455, 1983.

9. Anderson, R.N., and Rosenberg, H.M., Age standardisation of death rates: implementation of the year 2000 standard, *National Vital Statistics Reports*, 47(3), 1, 1998.

10. Miller, H.J., Tobler's first law and spatial analysis, *Annals of the Association of American Geographers*, 94(2), 284, 2004.

11. Openshaw, S., Charlton, A.W., Craft, M., and Birth, J.M., Preliminary communication: investigation of leukemia clusters by the use of a geographical analysis machine, *Lancet*, 1, 272, 1988.

12. Wakefield, S.E.L., Elliott, S.J., Cole, D.C., and Eyles, J.E., Environmental risk and (re)action: air quality, health, and civic involvement in an urban industrial neighbourhood, *Health & Place*, 7(3), 163, 2001.

13. Muehrcke, P.C., and Muehrcke, J.O., *Map Use — Reading, Analysis, and Interpretation*, 4th ed., JP Publications, Madison, WI, 1998.

14. Campbell, J., *Map Use and Analysis*, WCB/McGraw-Hill, Boston, MA, 2002.

15. Rushton, G., Improving the geographical basis of health surveillance using GIS, in *GIS and Health*, Gatrell, A.G., and Loytonen, M., Eds., Taylor & Francis, London, 1998, 65.

16. Gatrell, A.C., *Geographies of Health: An Introduction*, Blackwell, Oxford, 2002.

17. Staines, A., and Jarup, L., Health event data, in *Spatial Epidemiology: Methods and Applications*, Elliot, P., Wakefield, J.C., Best, N.G., and Briggs, D.J., Eds., Oxford University Press, Oxford, 2000, Chap. 2.

18. Dent, B.D., *Cartography: Thematic Map Design*, 3rd ed., Wm. C. Brown, Dubuque, IA, 1993.

19. Robinson, A.H., Morrison, J.L., Muehrcke, P.C., Kimerling, J., and Guptil, S., *Elements of Cartography*, 6th ed., Wiley, New York, NY, 1995.

20. Pyle, G.F., Introduction: foundations to medical geography, *Economic Geography*, 52, 95, 1976.

21. Pyle, G.F., *Applied Medical Geography*, Wiley, New York, NY, 1979.

22. Howe, G.M., *National Atlas of Disease Mortality in the United Kingdom*, T. Nelson, London, 1963.

23. McGalshan, N.D., *Medical Geography: Techniques and Field Studies*, Methuen, London, 1972.

24. Matheron, G., Principles of geostatistics, *Economic Geology*, 58, 1246, 1963.

25. Carrat, F., and Valleron, A.J., Epidemiologic mapping using the "kriging" method: application to an influenza-like illness epidemic in France, *American Journal of Epidemiology*, 135(11), 1293, 1992.

4

Point Pattern Methods of Disease Analysis

4.1 Examining Point Patterns

We established in Chapter 2 that the basic working units of disease data in a GIS include point (e.g., patient location), line (e.g., transmission route), and area (e.g., disease rate by county). Among these three data units, point data representing disease locations are the basic and most fundamental in spatial epidemiological studies. Point pattern analysis in spatial epidemiology concerns the distribution of disease events in space. At the elementary level, the spread of a disease in a community is revealed through the plotting of disease occurrences (at the residential locations of infected individuals) enabled with the geocoding or address matching function in a GIS (see Section 2.4 of Chapter 2 for detail). Point-by-point plotting is the simplest form of mapping disease occurrences.

A key question commonly raised is whether these disease occurrences and their spatial spread exhibit patterns of some sort (clustered, dispersed, or random). A simple means of exploring these concerns often involves a two-dimensional plot of the frequency distribution and making use of the Nearest Neighbour Index (NNI) to statistically analyze the intensity of the disease spread.[1] The method compares the average distance of the nearest other disease locations from each other (i.e., nearest neighbors) with a spatially random expected distance of the Poisson nature by dividing the empirical average nearest neighbor distance by the expected random distance to yield an NNI.

The values of NNI range between two theoretical extremes: 0 and 2.1491. The pattern represents the theoretical extreme of spatial concentration when all the points in a pattern fall at the same location, that is, the empirical nearest neighbor distance is 0 and NNI is 0. The more closely the points are clustered together, the closer to 0 NNI will be, because the average nearest neighbor distance decreases. The points are said to be randomly spaced when the NNI gets closer to 1. A pattern of perfectly uniformly spaced points is observed when NNI is equal to 2.1491. Accordingly, the closer NNI is to 2.1491, the more uniformly spaced the point distribution becomes.

NNI values may inwdicate for different spatial scales whether a disease pattern is clustered or dispersed. However, NNI alone is not sufficient in informing about the trend or the changing disease pattern over time. The locational shifts of disease hot spots over time represent an important concern in disease analysis. The Standard Deviational Ellipse (SDE) is a summary tool used to indicate an overall dispersion pattern and directional orientation.

Our investigative approach involves three stages, each with specific objectives and drawing on spatial analytical techniques of varying degrees of operational complexity. It is worth noting, as mentioned in Chapter 1, that this book is about methods to probe epidemiological data from the spatial perspective rather than trying to obtain answers about causes and risk factors of a disease. Following the footsteps of other researchers,[2,3] the three stages of analysis include the following: (1) elementary analysis involving simple visual inspection of a geographic phenomenon, (2) cluster analysis attempting the identification of possible hot spots, and (3) contextual analysis aiming to explain associative relationships between geographic phenomena.

Stage 1:   Elementary analysis of disease data by visualization

What was the distribution of severe acute respiratory syndrome (SARS) occurrences in Hong Kong? How should I interpret these maps? Where were the locations of both high- and low-frequency occurrences?

Stage 2:   Cluster analysis

Did the SARS occurrence exhibit a random distribution or a clustered pattern? How can we tell the intensity of spatial clustering?

Stage 3:   Contextual and geostatistical analysis

How could we describe the distributional patterns of SARS over time? Was it associated with specific social behaviors or environmental characteristics? How can we make use of the SDE in the analysis?

This chapter focuses on the methods and procedures of analyzing point data using partial data from the 2003 outbreak of SARS in Hong Kong (see Section 3.3 of Chapter 3 and Table B.2 of Appendix B for details of data composition). We start by conducting an elementary visual analysis using cartographic elements to identify the locations of disease concentration. Next, the degree of clustering is assessed, followed by a further examination of movement or the locational shifting of SARS over time using the SDE. The GIS software used in this chapter include GeoDa and CrimeStat (see Section 3.2.2 of Chapter 3 for instructions to download the software).

4.2 Elementary Analysis of Disease Data by Visualization

Objective:	To examine the spatial distribution of SARS occurrences
Software:	GeoDa and CrimeStat III
Epidemiological data:	SARS data of Hong Kong, April 1 to May 15, 2003 (Appendix B, Table B.2)
Boundary files:	Coastline and DC administrative boundaries of Hong Kong (Appendix B, Table B.6)
Spatial scale:	Hong Kong (DC districts)

Points to Consider

How would you describe the distribution of SARS disease occurrences in Hong Kong?

Step 1: Examining the SARS Data File

Table B.2 of Appendix B lists items or variables of the input data file in the DBF format. The residential buildings of individual SARS patients were recorded as the location of disease occurrences in three items: building name (B_NAME), block number (BLOCK), and street number (STREET). Before displaying these disease locations in a GIS, address matching was carried out to assign the x and y coordinates (X and Y) representing the centroids of residential buildings with persons infected with SARS. It should be noted that multiple occurrences of SARS patients residing in the same building will plot on top of each other, resulting in visual underrepresentation. This representational problem can be solved by using the kernel density method or by adding all occurrences of SARS of a building (CCOUNTS) to use the proportional symbol mapping technique (as shown in Figure 4.6).

Step 2: Reading Point Data into GeoDa

Invoke GeoDa and select "Tools > Shape > Points from DBF" to read data from a DBF file (Figure 4.1). Specify the labels of the columns containing the x and y coordinates and provide a name for your output SHP file. Click "Create" to start the process.

To display the x and y coordinates representing disease locations, select "File" and specify the name of the output SHP file from above (Figure 4.2). Specify REFNO as the key variable. Click "OK" to see the point distribution of disease cases.

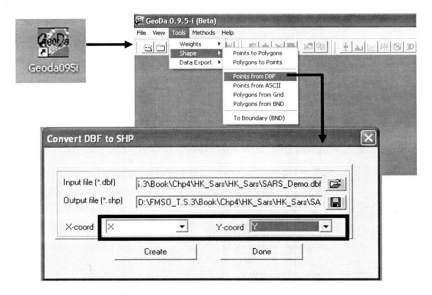

FIGURE 4.1
Reading point data into GeoDa.

Step 3: Adding a Base Map in GeoDa

Figure 4.2 shows the SARS cases without geographic features such as boundaries or roads to reference their positions. We will add a base map with district boundaries and the coastline of Hong Kong. Select the "Add Theme" icon and specify the name of the base map to load (Figure 4.3). Click "Open" to display disease cases on a base map.

    To improve visualization and readability, we may change the symbol color because the colors of points representing disease locations and the base map are very similar. Changing the color of a symbol or a group of symbols can be achieved by clicking on the respective color box under "Map Legend" in the map window (Figure 4.4).

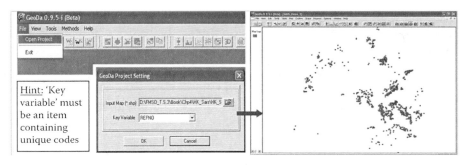

FIGURE 4.2
Displaying point data in GeoDa.

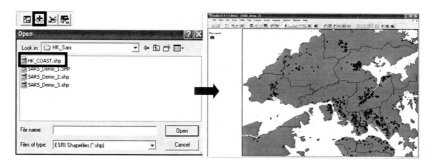

FIGURE 4.3
Displaying point data on a base map in GeoDa.

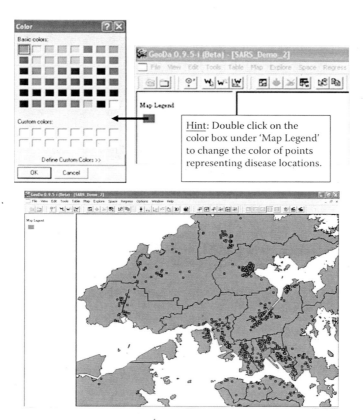

FIGURE 4.4
A color version of this figure follows page 108 Changing symbol color in GeoDa.

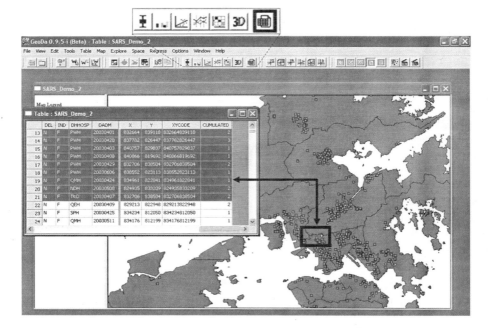

FIGURE 4.5
Linking map and attribute table in GeoDa. Select data records in the table and those selected are highlighted on the map and vice versa.

Step 4: Linking Interactively the Map and Its Disease Attribute Table

Select the icon representing an attribute table and a table will appear (Figure 4.5). Highlighting records in the attribute table will identify their corresponding locations on the map. Conversely, selecting a point or a group of points on the map will highlight the respective records in the table.

Points to Consider

Where were the locations of high-frequency occurrences?

Step 5: Displaying Disease Locations as Proportional Point Symbols

We made use of the HealthMapper to visualize locations of high disease occurrences (Figure 4.6). The HealthMapper supports a variety of mapping functions including the proportional point symbols, in which the sizes of circles are made to vary with magnitudes or disease counts at the corresponding locations. The proportional circle symbols displayed in Figure 4.6 are reflective of multiple occurrences in a building or some point locations.

At the initial level of surveillance, the spread of a disease in a community is revealed through the plotting of disease occurrences at the residential

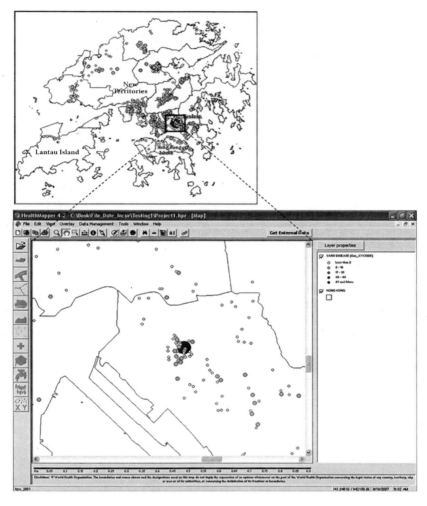

FIGURE 4.6
Displaying proportional circle symbols in HealthMapper. *Note:* The zoomed-in portion shows larger and darker circles in locations of higher disease occurrences.

addresses of infected persons enabled with the address matching function of a GIS. Point-by-point plotting is the simplest form of mapping disease occurrences for visualization, although proportional point symbols are more relevant for revealing not only positions but also magnitudes at the point locations. However, whether a disease pattern is clustered or dispersed can be rightly indicated by different measurements, for example, mode or nearest neighbor distance. Several typologies of cluster analysis have been developed because cluster routines typically fall into several general categories.[4] We will illustrate the procedures to undertake nearest neighbor analysis using CrimeStat.

4.3   Cluster Analysis: Nearest Neighbor Distance

Objective:	To examine the presence or absence of spatial clustering
Software:	GeoDa and CrimeStat III
Epidemiological data:	SARS data of Hong Kong, April 1 to May 15, 2003 (Table B.2 of Appendix B)
Boundary files:	Coastline and DC administrative boundaries of Hong Kong (Table B.6 of Appendix B)
Spatial scale:	Hong Kong (districts)

Points to Consider

Did the SARS occurrences exhibit a random distribution or a clustered pattern?

We will make use of the nearest neighbor analysis to examine possible patterns of spatial clustering of the SARS locations. The NNI measures the degree of spatial dispersion in the distribution based on the minimum interfeature distances or minimum distances between nearby points.[5] Small or near-zero NNI values indicate smaller distances between point features or a clustered pattern. NNI values in the vicinity of 1 indicate randomness, whereas larger values signify increased uniformity in point patterns.

Step 1: Setting Up a Workspace in CrimeStat

Activate the CrimeStat III program from the desktop or folder containing the installation file.

Step 2: Specifying Input Data

Figure 4.7 shows that the "Data Setup" tab in CrimeStat permits four types of input data: (1) primary file, (2) secondary file, (3) reference file, and (4) measurement parameters. Primary file refers to data of disease incidents (i.e., SARS in this case) that must contain the coordinate data of disease locations. CrimeStat can read many file formats: ASCII, DBF, SHP, DAT, MDB, and file formats conforming to the Open Data Base Connectivity (ODBC) standard interface.[6]

Users are required to indicate the columns containing coordinate information of the disease locations (i.e., X and Y in Table B.2 of Appendix B) and the coordinate system used. Given that the x and y coordinates are specified using the HK1980 grid system, the coordinate system is in "Projected (Euclidean)" and data units are in meters. If the coordinates come in longitudes and latitudes, then a spherical system is being used and data units will

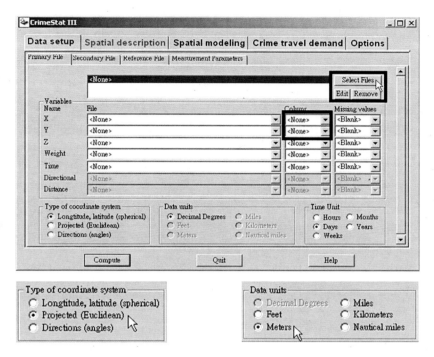

FIGURE 4.7
Specifying primary file input in CrimeStat.

automatically be in decimal places. For the projected coordinate systems, data units can be expressed in feet, meters, miles, and other. Time unit is not used in this section but will be used in Section 4.4.

Step 3: Specifying Measurement Parameters and Computing NNI

We will need to define "measurement parameters" to enable nearest neighbor analysis (Figure 4.8) by first specifying the areal coverage of the study area (e.g., the geographic coverage of Hong Kong = 1,078 km², or 1,078,000,000 m²) and the use of the "direct" method for distance measurement (see explanation box).

> **Explanation Box 4.1:** What are the types of distance measurement used in GIS? The direct method computes the shortest straight-line distance between two points on a surface of projected coordinates. Should a spherical coordinate system be adopted, the shortest distance between two points is a great circle arc. The indirect distance is an approximate measurement along a rectangular road network, whereas the network distance measures the actual driving distance along the network.

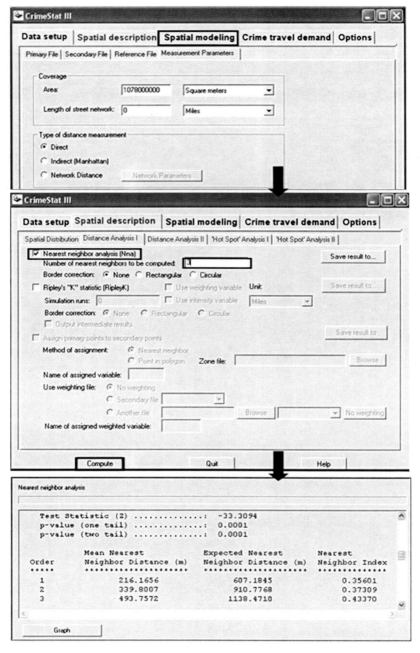

FIGURE 4.8
Nearest neighbor analysis in CrimeStat.

The NNI is one of the oldest distance statistics and an indicator of first-order spatial randomness because it compares the average distance of nearest neighbors against an expected random distance. In addition to a second- and third-order nearest neighbors, CrimeStat allows for the specification of *K*th-order NNI on the "Distance Analysis I" page, as illustrated in Figure 4.8.

The result of nearest neighbor analysis indicates that our SARS sample of 713 records exhibits a clustered pattern, with Z test statistics of −33.3094 significant at $p = .0001$ for both one- and two-tailed tests. The first-order clustering is obviously more compact (NNI = 0.35601) than the third-order clustering (NNI = 0.43370). Nonetheless, all three orders of nearest neighbors report NNI values closer to 0 than 1 and indicate a clustered pattern (Figure 4.9).

Step 4: Examining Local Patterns

The spatial scale to undertake a cluster analysis has a direct influence on its outcome. Given the results from Step 3 above, we shall now focus on Kwun Tong, a local community that reported a high concentration of SARS, to examine the applicability of the method. Obviously, we expect the NNI values to signify a strong presence of clusters because this community was the hardest hit during the outbreak. Having delimited the Kwun Tong district, we repeated Step 3 (above) to yield results in Figure 4.10.

Comparing Figures 4.9 and 4.10, we can see that both figures yield NNI values of less than 1, indicating the presence of clusters. However, clustering at the territorial scale, even with third-order neighbors (NNI = 0.43370), is more compact than observations made at the local scale (NNI for first-, second-, and third-order neighbors are 0.527, 0.605, and 0.629, respectively). These examples demonstrate that the NNI values vary with different spatial scales. From an epidemiological point of view, this inherent constraint of the nearest neighbor analysis inhibits its utility. Gatrell et al.[7] purported that kernel density estimation is of more value in estimating the intensity of one type of event relative to another. They pointed out that the kernel method can identify peaks that represent possible locations of clusters across a surface, or at least a subregion, worthy of further examination. We shall illustrate the kernel density method in Chapter 6.

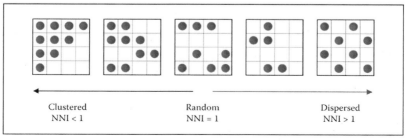

Clustered   Random   Dispersed
NNI < 1   NNI = 1   NNI > 1

FIGURE 4.9
Interpretation of the NNI.

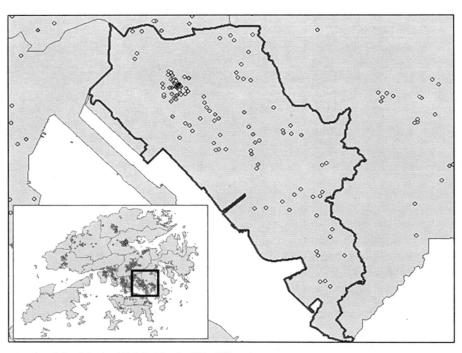

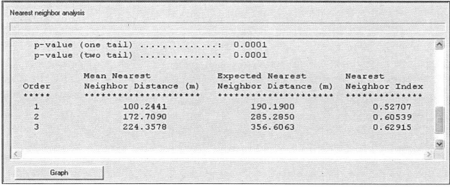

FIGURE 4.10
SARS occurrences in the district of Kwun Tong. Nearest neighbor analysis was done in CrimeStat, and results are displayed in HealthMapper.

4.4 Contextual Analysis

Objective:	To examine further the spatial spread of SARS over time
	Software: GeoDa and CrimeStat III
Epidemiological data:	A subset of SARS data of Hong Kong, April 1 to 5, 2003 (Table B.2 of Appendix B)
Boundary files:	Coastline and DC administrative boundaries of Hong Kong (Table B.6 of Appendix B)
Spatial scale:	Hong Kong (DC districts)

Points to Consider

Given daily accounts of disease data distributed over an area, how can we summarize these patterns over time?

We have seen from the preceding discussion that point patterns can be measured by using the — albeit scale-dependent — NNI. Are there methods besides the NNI that may be used to summarize the point patterns, particularly if there is a need to monitor these patterns over time? We know that standard deviation is a good statistical measure of the dispersion of data about the mean. In a two-dimensional space, we can show via a frequency histogram whether such a distribution is skewed in one direction or another. In a map representation, we can use SDE (see Explanation Box 4.2) as a means of summarizing the central tendency and dispersion in two dimensions, as well as indicating a directional trend.[8,9]

We extracted data for the first week of April 2003 to explore the directional trend and movement of SARS. In this demonstration, we considered the date in our database as the date of onset and assumed a five-day incubation period.[10] That is to say, a patient will appear in the database for five consecutive days from the date of onset.

Points to Consider

It is important in disease tracking and monitoring to record the date of onset (besides the date of admission) of a contagious individual.

Step 1: Setting Up a Workspace in CrimeStat

Activate CrimeStat III as described in Step 1 of Section 4.3.

Step 2: Specifying Input Data

The procedure is described in Step 2 of Section 4.3, but we will use a subset of the SARS data of Hong Kong (Table B.2 of Appendix B) as the input data. Each day under observation is a separate input file.

Explanation Box 4.2: What is an SDE? The SDE is derived from a bivariate distribution. There are two points of interest concerning the distribution of point locations across a two-dimensional space: (1) central tendency and (2) dispersion. As shown in the diagram below, the central tendency is the mean center and dispersion refers to the spread from the mean center as delimited by an ellipse. SDE is a graphic representation of standard deviation along the X and Y axes centered on the geometric mean of all locations. Its purpose is to provide a summary trend of the dispersion and examine whether a point distribution has a directional bias.

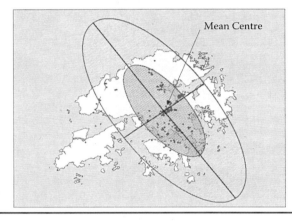

Mean Centre

N = 212
Standard Deviation Ellipses
Ellipse 1: x-length = 7889 m
             y-length = 18541 m
Ellipse 2: x-length = 15779 m
             y-length = 37082 m

Trend: NW-SE spread

Step 3: Specifying Measurement Parameters and Computing SDE

We checked the SDE to enable the function and specify "Save result to…" to the "Arcview SHP" format (Figure 4.11). The output for one day of observation is produced. Steps 2 and 3 are repeated for each day of the week under study, and the results are shown in Table 4.1. The figures for each day seem to vary from day to day but not by a substantial margin. We shall examine SDE in the graphic form next.

Step 4: Displaying SDE Using the HealthMapper

The HealthMapper is also used to examine results of the daily SDE. What may be inferred from the increasing size of the SDE from April 1 to April 5, 2003, is that the disease was spreading (Figure 4.12). The mean centers of these SDEs indicate the center of mass for each day. Tracking the movements and distances of these mean centers for successive days (Figure 4.13) may help provide advance warning about the direction and rate of disease spread. The northwest–southeast orientation of the ellipse indicates more spread in this direction, and the result seems to associate with the terrain (as constrained by water bodies toward the northeast and southwest of the ellipse) and settlement patterns.

Points to Consider

It is important to note that mean center is the arithmetic center of the point distribution. It may not necessarily locate in an area with disease incidence. For example, assuming the places of disease incidence are arranged in a circular structure, the mean center will be the middle of a circle with no reported cases.

The SDEs and their mean centers visually make explicit the spatial and temporal movements of a disease. Spatiotemporal analysis of disease estimates future disease patterns based on past trends. This method of disease tracking has implications for policy development and resource planning by alerting potential communities most at risk. The mapped results may also inform the development of illness prevention strategies based on seasonal, geographic, and population-specific demands, which we shall examine in Chapter 6.

SDEs can also be used to examine disease occurrences at the local scale. Figure 4.14 displays disease cases in the Shatin district, where the first case of SARS was recorded. A total of 263 occurrences were recorded within a period of 1.5 months (between April 1 and May 15, 2003). By specifying the minimum number of points per cluster in the "nearest neighbor hierarchical

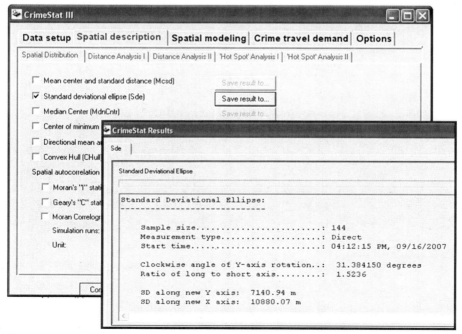

FIGURE 4.11
Output of SDE from CrimeStat.

TABLE 4.1

Results of SDEs for April 1 to 5, 2003

	April 1	April 2	April 3	April 4	April 5
Sample size	144	159	181	192	182
Clockwise angle of Y-axis rotation (°)	31.38	33.82	37.70	40.06	38.06
Ratio of the long to the short axis after rotation	1.52	1.49	1.57	1.60	1.63
Standard deviation along the new X axes (m)	10,880.07	11,227.79	11,303.66	11,559.41	11,671.48
Standard deviation along the new Y axes (m)	7,140.94	7,522.67	7,199.13	7,202.82	7,145.84
X-axes length	21,760.14	22,455.57	22,607.32	23,118.82	14,291.68
Y-axes length	14,281.88	15,045.33	14,398.27	14,405.65	23,342.96
Area of the ellipse defined by these axes (km²)	244.083	265.348	255.652	261.570	262.017
Standard deviation along the X axes	21,760.14	22,455.57	22,607.32	23,118.82	23,342.96
Standard deviation along the Y axes	14,281.88	15,045.33	14,398.27	14,405.65	14,291.68
X-axes length for a 2× SDE	43,520.29	44,911.14	45,214.65	46,237.64	46,685.92
Y-axes length for a 2× SDE	28,563.75	30,090.66	28,796.54	28,811.29	28,583.36
Area of the 2× ellipse defined by these axes (km²)	976.331	1,061.392	1,022.608	1,046.281	1,048.067

spatial clustering" function, CrimeStat allows the computation of SDEs for a selected region. SDEs of a smaller size tend to indicate compactness of disease concentration. This tool not only summarizes disease clustering within a district but also pinpoints possible problem areas (or housing estates in this case) for targeted intervention measures.

4.5   Constraints and Limitations

Point data represent the most detailed account of an epidemiological event, but such spatial characterization may be simplistic or even misleading. We

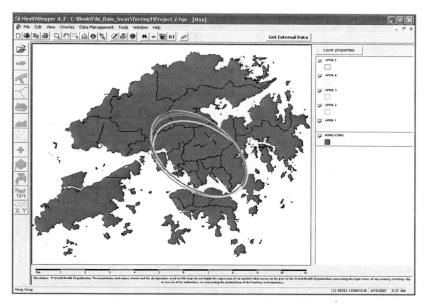

FIGURE 4.12
A color version of this figure follows page 108 Displaying results of SDE in the HealthMapper.

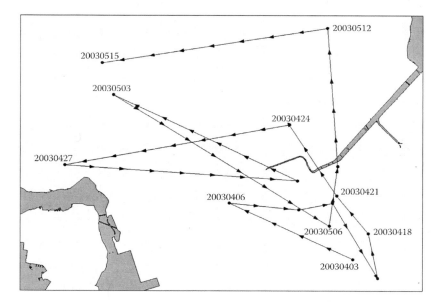

FIGURE 4.13
Displaying results of SDE in the HealthMapper. A plot of the mean centers of daily SDE of SARS occurrences from April 3 to May 15, 2003, reveals mingling of the disease concentration in Tai Wai and its neighboring areas (as indicated by the looping tracks) and a northward then westward progression toward Kwai Chung in the later part of the epidemic.

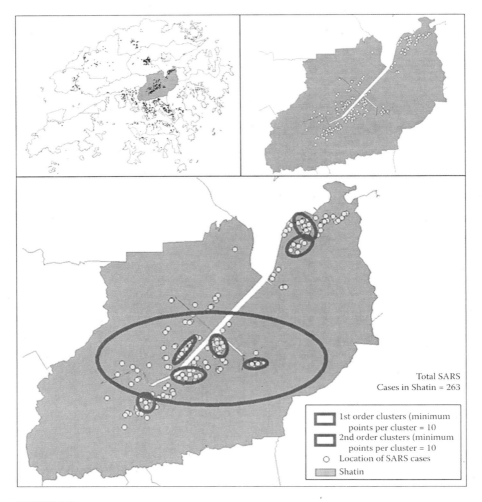

FIGURE 4.14

SARS clusters in the Shatin district of Hong Kong, April 1 to May 15, 2003. SDEs were done in CrimeStat, and results are displayed in HealthMapper.

based our analysis of disease incidence by reducing the spatial existence of individuals to a single point, using their home addresses. This assumption is grossly deficient because disease transmission can happen at work, school, or any other venue, which can be far from the home. Lai et al.[10] showed that there were pockets of non-residential nosocomial infections besides community clusters of superspreading events during the 2003 SARS outbreak in Hong Kong.

Furthermore, the level of characterization available from point patterns is rather limited, given that only two properties can be consistently measured.

These are measures of density and distance, both computed using standard nearest neighbor and linear distance methods. Our demonstrations also illustrate that point pattern analysis is very sensitive to the definition of the study area because a regularly distributed pattern can be made to appear clustered by including large margins around the study area. These measures are also subject to boundary corrections, and most often, study area boundaries have to be redefined to become a convex polygon over the study area or, in the simplest form, as rectangles bounding the points under analysis.

4.6 Summary

We have introduced some of the key procedures to undertake point pattern analysis in health studies using GeoDa and CrimeStat. It is of course always important to plot the point events to visually detect the outliers. When the number of points becomes overwhelmingly large to handle, we may use appropriate tools (such as SDE) to summarize the observations. In the next chapter, we will examine how we can conduct a more informed spatial analysis based on point and areal (enumerated census) data.

References

1. Taylor, P.J., *Quantitative Methods in Geography — An Introduction to Spatial Analysis*, Houghton Mifflin, Hopewell, NJ, 1977.
2. Bailey, T.C., and Gatrell, A.C., *Interactive Spatial Data Analysis*, Longman, Harlow, 1995.
3. Olson, J., A coordinate approach to map communication improvement, *The American Cartographer*, 3(2), 151, 1976.
4. Everett, B., *Cluster Analysis*, Heinemann Educational Books, London, 1974.
5. Chou, Y.H., *Exploring Spatial Analysis in Geographic Information Systems*, OnWord Press, Santa Fe, NM, 1997.
6. Levine, N., *CrimeStat 1.1, A Spatial Statistics Program for the Analysis of Crime Incident Locations*, National Institute of Justice, Washington, DC, 2000.
7. Gatrell, A.C., Bailey, T.C., Diggle, P.J., and Rowlingson, B.S., Spatial point pattern analysis and its application in geographical epidemiology, *Transactions of the Institute of British Geographers*, 21(1), 256, 1996.
8. Ebdon, D., *Statistics in Geography*, 2nd ed., with corrections, Blackwell, Oxford, 1988.
9. Cromley, R.G., *Digital Cartography*, Prentice Hall, Englewood Cliffs, NJ, 1992.

10. Lai, P.C., Wong, C.M., Hedley, A.J., Lo, S.V., Leung, P.Y., Kong, J., and Leung, G.M., Understanding the spatial clustering of severe acute respiratory syndrome (SARS) in Hong Kong, *Environmental Health Perspectives*, 112(15), 1550, 2004.

5

Areal Methods of Disease Analysis

5.1   Areal Pattern Analysis

A fundamental issue concerning spatial epidemiology is how the disease data have been observed or sampled. The method of data collection can have a great impact on the results. In many occasions, the exact positions of disease incidence at the street address level may not be known and only statistics at the census tract level are available (e.g., changwat or province in Thailand and DC districts in Hong Kong). Even under situations where exact locations are known, grouped or aggregated data are preferred for reasons of data privacy and ease of interpretation (see Section 2.5 of Chapter 2). The use of count models allows point-based data to be aggregated based on some areal units or census tracts.

Areal-based or choropleth mapping is one technique to deal with overlapping point symbols in visualizing disease data on maps. It is a conventional method of summarizing spatial data based on statistical, administrative, or enumeration units. Each enumeration unit is colored, shaded, dotted, or hatched on a choropleth such that the colors are graded in proportion to the varying magnitudes of a variable. Simply put, disease clusters can be understood as an enumeration area with a high frequency of disease incidents. A convenient method of identifying hot spots is to partition the jurisdiction into fixed enumeration units and develop a set of data classification rules using predefined threshold values.[1]

5.2   Areal Mapping

5.2.1   Disease Rates

Aim:	To undertake the calculation of disease rate of dengue by two different administrative boundaries of Thailand and present them as choropleth maps
Objective:	Exploring disease rate mapping and functions of GeoDa Software: Microsoft Excel and GeoDa
Epidemiological data:	Suspected dengue cases of Thailand in 2004 (Table B.3 of Appendix B)
Boundary files:	Administrative boundary data of province (changwat) and district (amphoe) of Thailand (Tables B.7 and B.8 of Appendix B)
Spatial scale:	Thailand (province and district)

A very important step before doing areal-based mapping is to summarize the point data by different administrative boundaries. Summarization can be done in two ways depending on the attribute data available:

i. Use the "point-in-polygon" method, that is, overlay the polygon file of an administrative boundary over data on disease incidence to undertake counting by area.

ii. Summarize the point data in Excel if zoning data (i.e., codes of an administrative boundary) are available in the attribute table.

The first method makes use of the point-in-polygon function, which is usually not available in GIS freeware; however, this function is found in almost all commercial GIS. The procedure to summarize point data by districts using the second method is described in Appendix C.

Assuming that data on areal-based counts are available, the following section demonstrates the steps to create a disease rate map in GeoDa (see Section 3.2.2 of Chapter 3 for procedures to install the software).

1. Start GeoDa by double clicking on the program icon.

2. Choose "File > Open Project," and specify a data layer (e.g., dengue counts by province of Thailand). Locate the file path where the data layer is stored, and select a unique identifier (such as a record identifier) as the "Key Variable."

3. Choose "Map > Smooth > Raw Rate > Quantile" and 5 for "# of Classes/Groups" to plot disease rates by the enumeration units.

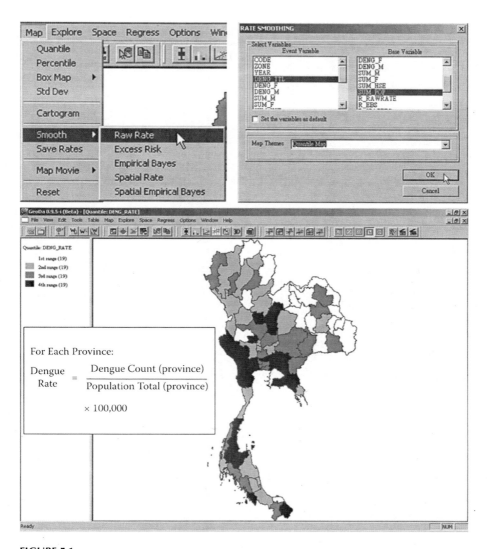

FIGURE 5.1
A map of dengue rate per 100,000 population by province in Thailand using the quantile method in GeoDa.

Figure 5.1 shows the use of DENG_TOL as the event variable and the total population SUM_POP as the base variable to compute the dengue rate. Given that raw rates yield very small numbers, they were converted to rates per 100,000 population before mapping.

Points to Consider

The steps above may be repeated for another layer of administrative boundary (e.g., district or amphoe as in Figure 5.2). Which of the two maps is more meaningful and why?

4. Select "Map > Std Dev" to create another map using a different classification method by standard deviation (Figure 5.3).

Points to Consider

How does Figure 5.3 (by standard deviation) compare with Figure 5.2 (by quantile)? Would you consider Figure 5.3 easier or more difficult to interpret? Are there similarities or differences?

5. Select "Explore > Histogram" to reveal the frequency distribution by data classes (Figure 5.4).
6. Save the disease rate (i.e., dengue counts/total population) in a new column by right-clicking on the map and choosing "Save Rates" (Figure 5.5).

5.2.2   Rate Smoothing Techniques

Many applications in epidemiological or other studies use rates to estimate the underlying risk. However, extreme values in the population distribution may result in variance instability and outliers in the raw rates. Rate smoothing is one solution to deal with such variance instability by borrowing strengths from other spatial units. More detailed discussion on rate smoothing is available at the GeoDa homepage (www.geoda.uiuc.edu/support/help/glossary.html#smooth).

5.2.2.1   *The Empirical Bayes Smoothing Method*

The empirical Bayes (EB) smoothing method calculates a raw rate for each areal unit averaged against a separately computed reference estimate based on the whole study region, such as the overall population mean. This statistical smoother is used to correct for the variance instability associated with rates that have a small base.

1. Select "Map > Smooth > Empirical Bayes" to use the selected smoothing method on a new map (Figure 5.6b).

5.2.2.2   *The Spatial Empirical Bayes Smoothing Method*

The spatial empirical Bayes (SEB) smoothing method differs from EB smoothing in that the correction for variance instability is localized as opposed to global (i.e., based on all observations). Unlike the use of a constant mean and

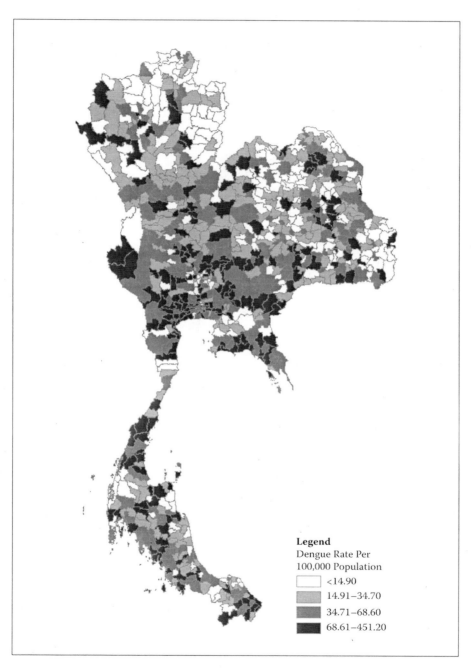

FIGURE 5.2
A map of dengue rate by district in Thailand using the quantile method in GeoDa.

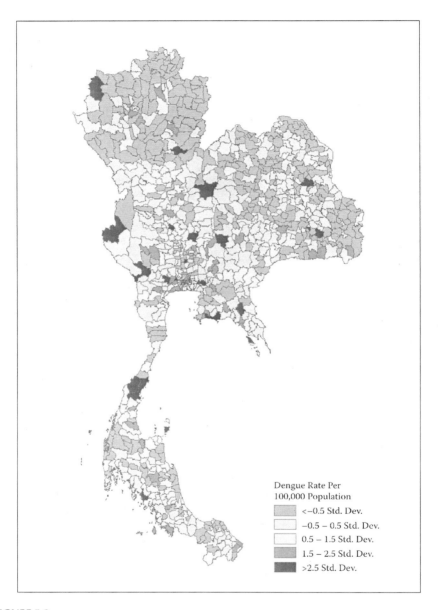

FIGURE 5.3
A color version of this figure follows page 108 A map of dengue rate by province in Thailand using the standard deviation method in GeoDa.

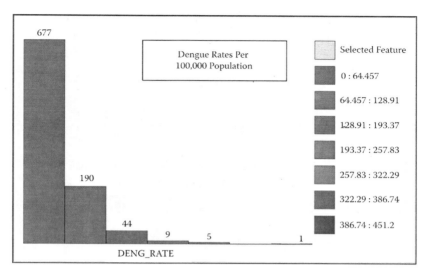

FIGURE 5.4
A frequency histogram of dengue rates used in Figure 5.2.

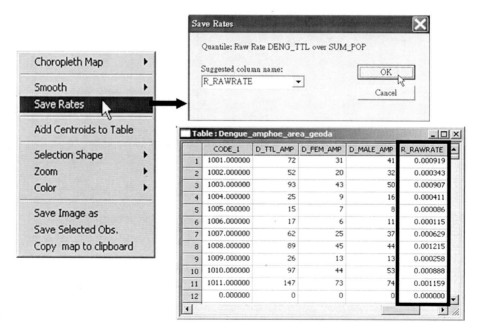

FIGURE 5.5
Saving a column of computed rates in GeoDa.

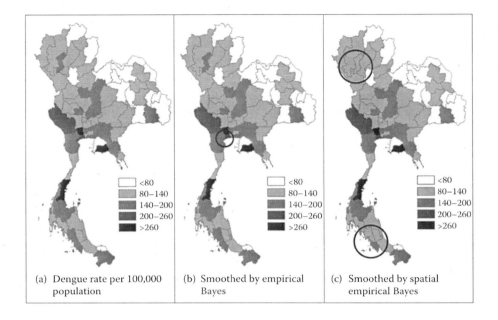

(a) Dengue rate per 100,000 population

(b) Smoothed by empirical Bayes

(c) Smoothed by spatial empirical Bayes

FIGURE 5.6
Maps of dengue rate by province in Thailand using different smoothers in GeoDa.

variance in the regular EB case, the SEB smoother is based on a locally vary-ing reference mean and variance.

1. Select "Tools > Weights > Create" to create a spatial weight file (.gwt). The weights file is required for the computation of spatial autocor-relation statistics and implementation of the SEB smoothing method. It is actually a matrix of spatial weights constructed by considering contiguity between polygons or areal units and the spatial separa-tion between them.

2. In the "Creating Weights" dialog, locate the input file and specify the path for the output file. Then select "an ID variable for the weights file" or leave the option as default. Choose "Queen Contiguity" (see Explanation Box 5.1) from the tab and use default options for the rest (Figure 5.6c).

3. Save the EB and the SEB rates by right-clicking on the respective maps in GeoDa. Choose "Save Rates > OK" to accept the suggested column name. The saved columns are appended at the end of the attribute table.

Explanation Box 5.1: What is meant by spatial contiguity? Spatial contiguity is a measure to check for continuity between areas (i.e., whether the polygons share a border). This neighbor relationship can loosely represent a measure of potential interaction between adjoining areas. Three types of contiguity from the center cell are possible: rook, bishop, and queen.

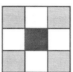

Rook Neighbours   Bishop Neighbours   Queen Neighbours

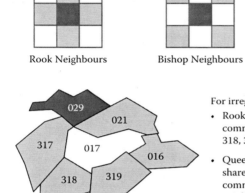

For irregular units:

- Rook neighbours of 017 share common borders (e.g., 317, 318, 319, 016, 021)

- Queen neighbours of 017 share common vertex and common borders (e.g., all rook neighbours plus 029)

Rook contiguity uses only common boundaries to define neighbors, whereas queen contiguity includes all common points (boundaries and vertices) in the definition. Therefore, spatial weights based on the queen contiguity always have a denser connectedness given more neighbors. Only rook and queen contiguities are available in GeoDa. The queen contiguity is adopted in disease surveillance studies because disease infection is usually not directional restricted.

Points to Consider

Compare rate maps in Figures 5.2 and 5.6. Can you explain the difference between the maps? Which one do you prefer?

5.3   Constraints and Limitations of Choropleth Mapping

5.3.1   Data Classification in Choropleth Maps

The choropleth method has obvious deficiencies in its visualization. These concerns arise from data classification, which may not only mislead interpretation but also hide the true message behind a distributional pattern. For instance, the rate of a disease infection using raw population total as the denominator will be significantly different from that of the number of dwelling units. Figure 5.7 displays the locations of dengue incidents and the dengue rate per 100,000 individuals at the district level in Bangkok, using five different methods of data classification for five distinct classes in each case:

1. Natural break: Gaps or depressions are used to draw boundaries between classes.
2. Equal area: Classes are separated based on the equality of area.
3. Equal interval: Classes are separated into sectors of equal range determined by dividing the data range by the number of sectors.
4. Equal count (quantile): Values are ordered and separated into classes containing approximately the same number of observations.
5. Standard deviation: Classes are divided based on a statistical measure of data distribution around the mean.

The rate maps by districts in Bangkok in Figure 5.7 show the locations of dengue reports overlaid on the same area. Although the dengue cases and the population for each district have remained constant, the underlying choropleth patterns displaying the rates on these five maps are quite different because of the different classification methods. For instance, pockets of districts in the central location exhibit a higher incidence rate on maps B and D but show variable readings on maps C and E. The choice of a suitable classification method clearly affects the impression conveyed.

Figure 5.8 displays histograms of the dengue rates shown on maps A to E in Figure 5.7. The dotted horizontal lines on the histograms indicate the class breaks, and the gray bars indicate the limits or data range of the five classes. All histograms in Figure 5.8 are alike, but the use of five different classification methods obviously yields distinctively different divisions of classes.

The data range of each class is unequal in the natural break classification (A) because the class breaks occur at gaps in the data set. The number of districts falling in the middle three classes is nearly the same because of little variation in the data set. In contrast, few cases fall in the highest and lowest classes because of a small number of extreme values in the data. The natural break classification is useful in highlighting areas of extreme differences because the degree of data variation is considered.

The equal area (B) and quantile (D) options are rather similar classification methods in which an approximate number of observations is assigned to each class. A major difference between the two is the size consideration of areas in the equal area method. Because the study area has relatively fewer areas of small sizes, the number of districts belonging to the two lowest classes is fewer for the equal area method (B). In general, the two methods are preferred in situations where values are not in the extreme ranges because of

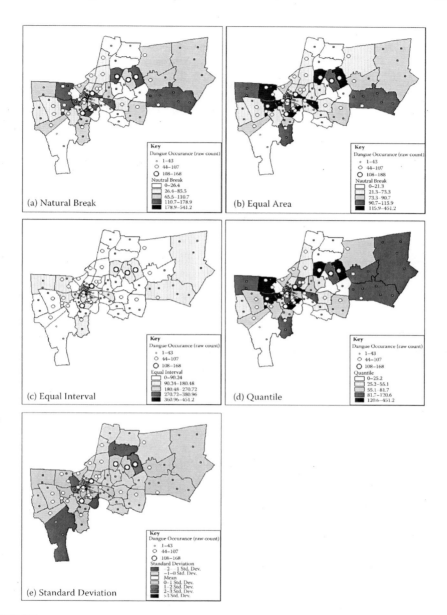

FIGURE 5.7
A color version of this figure follows page 108 Maps of dengue rates per 100,000 population in Bangkok using different classification methods.

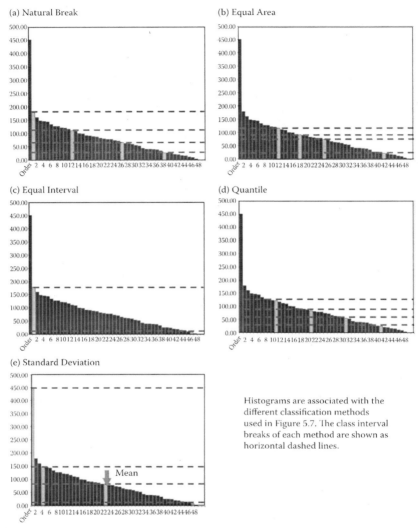

FIGURE 5.8
Histograms of dengue rates by different classification methods shown in Figure 5.7.

the possibility of exaggerating the degree of a phenomenon at both ends (see maps B and D in Figure 5.7).

The equal interval classification (C) subdivides data into classes of equal range. This method tends to favor low values and underestimates the degree of seriousness of a phenomenon. A similar situation is found in the case of standard deviation classification (E), which is effective in illustrating data distribution about the mean. This method replaces numerical values with statistical classes to indicate the degree of variation of an area from the mean, which is considered the norm.

The matter of data classification in choropleth mapping is further complicated by the number of classes and the class intervals. A number of suggestions have been made by researchers in this regard. Unwin[2] suggested four to eight classes in one map, although modern computers can support colors in the millions. Although the choice of class interval class depends on a multitude of factors (including data size, intended message presented, frequency distribution of the phenomenon, and size of the study area), Evans[3] suggested that standard deviation intervals could be used if data were normally distributed, whereas regular intervals would be more suitable for data of more uniform distribution.

5.3.2 Modifiable Areal Unit and Area Dependence Problems

The presence of variations in the modeling result arising from aggregating data by different enumeration units is known as the MAUP in geography (see Section 2.5 of Chapter 2). MAUP is a classical problem in choropleth mapping where the delineation of hot spots or areas of high incidence is distorted by natural boundaries and artificial features that break up the populated areas.[4]

Individual incidents are obviously subject to certain degrees of generalization after agglomeration based on the measurement scale of the enumeration units. Because such a measurement scale is a matter of choice, one can easily remove apparent patterns through different data classifications of the mapped variable. It is also equally possible to design zoning divisions that exaggerate high frequencies of a phenomenon. This area dependence effect is illustrated in Figure 5.9 using the Pearson product-moment correlation coefficient (r) from conventional statistical analysis.[2]

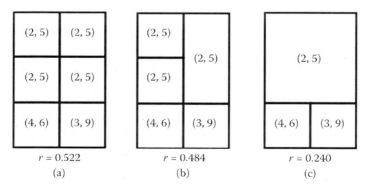

Grid cells of regular and equal sizes are used in this example. The numbers shown in the cells represent density values of two variables x and y.

FIGURE 5.9
Area dependence problem. (Adapted from Unwin.[2])

Figure 5.9a shows four of the six zones having the same (x and y) readings with an r coefficient of 0.522. Figure 5.9b combines two of the zones into one, but its r value of 0.484 differs slightly from that in Figure 5.9a, although the two constructs are basically the same. The difference becomes more apparent in Figure 5.9c, where the r value is reduced to 0.240 when four zones of similar readings are aggregated. The illustrations serve to explain that the imposition of different enumeration units could lead to totally different results whatever the underlying true correlation may be, and the disparity could be worse with areas of irregular shapes.

5.4   Spatial Dependence

Spatial dependency concerns the covariation of characteristics within a geographic space. A phenomenon may show no specific patterns of association with space (i.e., random) or appear to be correlated either positively or negatively. In the case of a spatial association, we may wish to find out whatever is causing an observation in a location to be similar or dissimilar to its nearby locations.

There are three possible explanations for these situations: (1) simple correlation, (2) causal relationship, and (3) spatial interaction. In the first instance, disease rates in a community tend to be similar to socioeconomic status (measured by median income and/or educational attainment), increasing or decreasing the likelihood for that type of disease. Another possibility is that an incident at a given location is directly influenced by something in the nearby locations. For example, the locations of falls suggest the presence of certain environmental characteristics (uneven pavement, slippery walkway, busy intersection, poor lighting, etc.) causing the increased incidence rate. Finally, the movement of people and goods creates opportunities for the apparent relationships between locations. Individuals infected with a contagious disease are likely to transmit the disease to people at home, work, or other key locations of the subject's activities.

In statistical terms, spatial autocorrelation means that the value of a variable is associated with the values on the same variable in nearby or adjacent polygons. It is the correlation of a variable with itself through space. There are associated measures to test the level of interdependence among the variables, the nature, and strength of the interdependence. These diagnostic tools will be used to determine if there is spatial autocorrelation and, if so, whether the relationship is positive or negative.

Points to Consider

Why is spatial autocorrelation important? Most statistics are based on the assumption that the values of observations in each sample are independent of each other. A positive spatial autocorrelation may violate this, if the samples were taken from nearby areas. The goal of spatial autocorrelation is to measure the strength of spatial association in a map and test the assumption of independence or randomness.

5.4.1 Measures of Spatial Autocorrelation

Spatial autocorrelation measures the extent to which an occurrence in space (whether point or area) is similar to or unlike occurrences in a neighboring areal unit. It is computed by dividing the spatial covariation by the total variation. In the case of raster data, neighbors are determined on an eight-directional queen case or the nondiagonal, four-directional rook case (see Explanation Box 5.1 about spatial contiguity). Popular measures of spatial autocorrelation with spatial analysis include indices such as Moran's *I* and Geary's *C* (see also Section 3.4.3 of Chapter 3).

Moran's *I* is one of the oldest indicators of spatial autocorrelation.[5] It is a popular measure and has remained a de facto standard in examining zones or points with continuous variables associated with them. Moran's *I* is similar to the Pearson's correlation coefficient and gives a score ranging between –1 and 1. A positive score means a "hot" spot or that a polygon or point with a high score has other polygons or points with high scores surrounding it. Conversely, an occurrence of a low score indicates a "cold" spot because of low scoring occurrences in the neighborhood. A score of zero indicates that nothing can be assumed about the scores of the neighboring polygons or points. A negative score means a "spatial outlier" or that the scores of neighboring locations will be the opposite of the location under examination; that is, a polygon or point with a low score will have high scoring neighbors, and vice versa.

Geary's *C* is a statistical technique similar but inversely related to Moran's *I* in assessing the degree of spatial autocorrelation present in the data.[6] It does not provide identical inference because it emphasizes the difference in values between pairs of observations as opposed to the covariation between the pairs. The Moran coefficient gives a more global indicator, whereas Geary's *C* is more sensitive to differences in small neighborhoods. Geary's *C* values typically range between 0 and 2, but values greater than 2 can occasionally be found.[7] A score of zero indicates a strong positive spatial autocorrelation to 2, which represents a strong negative spatial autocorrelation.

Although the strength of Moran's coefficient lies in its simplicity, its major limitation is the tendency to average local variations in situations of spatial autocorrelation. The LISA[8,9] can be seen as the local equivalent of Moran's *I*

For each location, LISA values allow for the computation of its similarity with its neighbors and also to test its significance. Five scenarios may emerge:

▪	High-high	**Hot spots** or locations with high values with similar neighbors
▪	Low-low	**Cold spots** or locations with low values with similar neighbors
▪	Low-high	Potential **spatial outliers** or locations with low values with high-value neighbors
▪	High-low	Potential **spatial outliers** or locations with high values with low-value neighbors
☐	Not Significant	Locations with **no significant local autocorrelation**

FIGURE 5.10
A color version of this figure follows page 108 Local indicators of spatial association.

in showing hot and cold spots (clusters of high and low scores, respectively) as well as spatial outliers (where there is a mixture of high and low scores in neighboring areas) (Figure 5.10).

5.5   Spatial Autocorrelation Analysis with GeoDa

Objective:	To examine spatial autocorrelation of dengue occurrences Software: GeoDa (see Anselin[9])
Epidemiological data:	Suspected dengue cases in 2004 (Appendix B, Table B.3)
Boundary files:	Coastline and administrative boundaries of Thailand (Appendix B, Tables B.7 and B.8)
Spatial scale:	Thailand (province and district)

Points to Consider

Was the distribution of dengue disease occurrences spatially correlated?

Step 1: Examining the Dengue Data File

Table B.3 in Appendix B lists items or variables of the dengue cases in the DBF format. The villages of individual dengue patients were recorded as the locations of disease occurrences, along with their associated subdistricts, districts, and provinces. The demonstration below makes use of data at the changwat or province level that have predefined X and Y coordinate pairs for the polygon centroids (Table B.8 in Appendix B).

It should be noted that multiple occurrences of dengue patients residing in the same province will be plotted on top of each other, resulting in visual underrepresentation. There is a need here to aggregate and count occurrences of dengue by the 76 provinces. Add a column of dengue counts to the changwat boundary data (Table B.8 in Appendix B) to record the total dengue cases by province. We have illustrated (in Step 5 of Section 4.2 of Chapter 4) the proportional symbol mapping technique to represent count data by areal units.

The procedures for spatial autocorrelation analysis are structured (see Explanation Box 5.2). We shall use the univariate method for investigating dengue occurrences per 100,000 population or DENG_RATE at the provincial level.

Explanation Box 5.2: Steps in examining spatial autocorrelation. Spatial autocorrelation analysis in GeoDa can be conducted on univariate, bivariate, or standardized rate variables. In the univariate case, spatial autocorrelation compares the value of a variable at a location (e.g., disease incidence) against the weighted value of the same variable for all neighboring locations. In the bivariate case, the value of a variable at a location (e.g., disease incidence) is compared against the weighted value of a different variable (e.g., population) or the same variable for different periods at neighboring locations. Standardized rate variables are values that have been adjusted (e.g., age-adjusted mortality rate or z score). A sequence of seven steps in spatial autocorrelation is summarized in the table below.

Steps	Description	Functions
1	Examine data	Inspect data and select variable(s)
2	Establish spatial weights	Record information about neighborhood structure for each location (considering first-order contiguity only)
3	Examine characteristics of spatial weights	Use a histogram of observations ordered by the numbers of neighbors to check for unconnected observations
4	Compute spatial lags	Spatial lags is the sum of weighted values of neighboring locations around a central location
5	Visualize Moran scatterplot	Study the standardized plot of the original variable against the spatial lags for clusters or outliers
6	Compute statistical significance	Assess the significance of the Moran's I statistic against a null hypothesis of no spatial autocorrelation
7	Compile LISA	Assess the local version of Moran's I to see how spatial autocorrelation varies over the region

Step 2: Constructing Spatial Weights

Select Tools > Weights > Create or click on the "Create Weights" icon to construct a spatial weight file to record information about the neighborhood structure for each location (Figure 5.11). GeoDa offers several methods to create spatial weights but we will use simple first-order queen contiguity weights.

Specify in ❶ names of input (a shapefile) and output (the spatial weights) files as well as a unique variable or identifier for the areal units. Select in ❷ the type of spatial contiguity (rook or queen) on which to compute the weights. Define in ❸ the method of distance computation and variables that store *X* and *Y* coordinates of the polygon centroids.

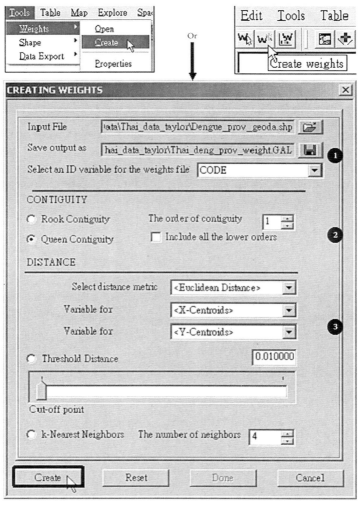

FIGURE 5.11
Constructing spatial weights in GeoDa.

Step 3: Examining Characteristics of Spatial Weights

A histogram showing the distribution of observations according to how many neighbors they have can be obtained by selecting Tools > Weights > Properties or by clicking on the "Weights Characteristics" toolbar (Figure 5.12). It is usually a good practice to check the characteristics of the spatial weights file to identify undesirable characteristics (such as outliers) of the data set.

Step 4: Constructing Spatially Lagged Variables

A "spatially lagged variable" is the sum of weighted values of neighboring locations around a central location (Figure 5.13). A new column in the attribute table is needed to store the computed spatially lagged values. Make sure the spatial weight file from Step 3 is open. Next, open the attribute table of the input shapefile, right-click to select "Add Column," and name the new column SPAT_LAG. Right-click on the attribute table again to select "Field Calculation." Select "Lag Operations," and specify SPAT_LAG as the result. Make sure the correct weights file is specified, and choose DENG_RATE as the variable to use.

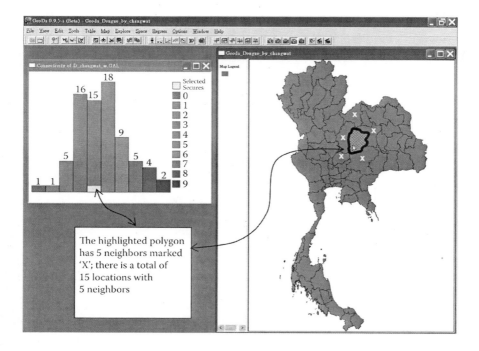

FIGURE 5.12
Examining characteristics of spatial weights in GeoDa.

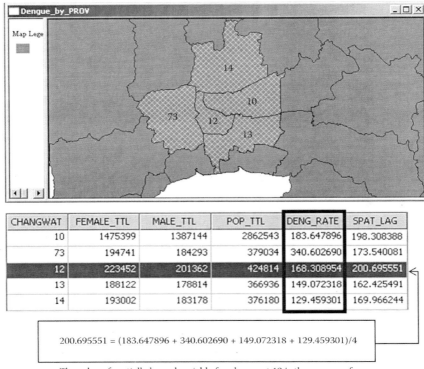

$$200.695551 = (183.647896 + 340.602690 + 149.072318 + 129.459301)/4$$

The value of spatially lagged variable for changwat 12 is the average of the sum of dengue rate of neighbors in changwat 10, 73, 13, and 14.

FIGURE 5.13
Computation of a spatially lagged variable in GeoDa.

Step 5: Visualizing the Moran Scatterplot

Select "Space > Univariate Moran," and choose DENG_RATE as the first variable under "Variables Settings." Then select the proper spatial weight file (with GAL extension), and click "OK" to continue. The Moran scatterplot in Figure 5.14 shows the Moran's I statistics of 0.2035 ($p = .0040$), which is the slope of the regression line. The four quadrants in the scatterplot correspond to different types of spatial autocorrelation as indicated (see also Figure 5.10).

The various categories of clusters (hot spots, cold spots, and outliers) in the Moran scatterplot can be examined visually by clicking the respective quadrants. The corresponding observations (i.e., provinces or changwat) falling in each category will be highlighted in the map display for visual inspection.

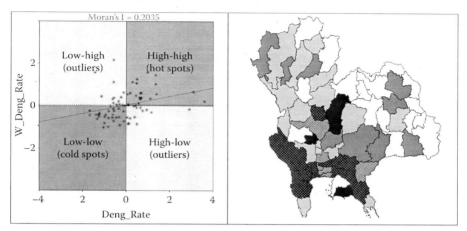

Note: Highlighting the first quadrant on the scatter plot (left) reveals provinces belonging to the 'High-high' (hot spots) category (right)

FIGURE 5.14
A color version of this figure follows page 108 A Moran scatterplot in GeoDa.

Step 6: Assessing Statistical Significance of Moran's *I*

The significance of Moran's *I* statistics is assessed against the null hypothesis of no spatial autocorrelation using the permutation procedure in GeoDa. Select "Options > Randomization > 999 Permutations" to generate a reference distribution (Figure 5.15). A *p* value of .004 in this case indicates that the null hypothesis is rejected and that there is positive spatial autocorrelation (Moran's *I* = 0.2035) for the dengue rates of Thailand.

We can turn on the "Envelope Slopes" option to indicate the 5th and 95th percentiles in the reference distribution under spatial randomness (Figure 5.15). The plot indicates possible regions where the spatial autocorrelation may be different from the rest. Specifically, points inside the envelope on the scatterplot have Moran's *I* values in the lower 5th or upper 95th range, suggesting little or no spatial autocorrelation for these observations.

Step 7: Compiling Univariate LISA

The univariate LISA statistics are obtained by selecting "SPACE > Univariate LISA" and indicating DENG_RATE as the first variable. This option generates four graphs as indicated in Figure 5.16. Map (a) shows the LISA clusters significant at *p* = .01 and interpreted as explained in Figure 5.10. Each colored cluster matches a quadrant of the Moran scatterplot in graph (d). Map (b) is a Moran significance map differentiated by different significance levels (*p* = .05, *p* = .01, *p* = .001, and *p* = .0001) indicated in different shades of green. Graph (c) is a box plot showing the distribution of individual LISA statistics.

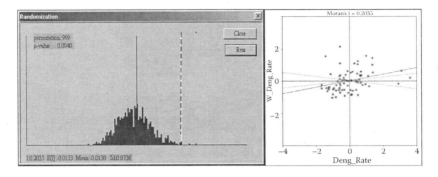

FIGURE 5.15

A reference distribution (left) and Moran scatterplot showing the 5th and 95th percentiles (right) in GeoDa.

The goal of spatial autocorrelation is to measure the strength of spatial association in a region and test the assumption of independence or randomness. Homogeneity cannot be assumed if spatial autocorrelation exists. The test draws our attention to the presence of hot and cold spots but does not explain why. For example, could the presence of dengue cold spots in the northeastern part of Thailand (see map [a] in Figure 5.16) be related to topography (high hills and mountains) and climate (wintry and foggy)? There is a need to undertake further analysis about the circumstances and conditions that surround an event.

5.6   Summary

It is considered too confidential by most governments to use data at the individual household level in the census. Some form of enumeration units of assumed uniformity (e.g., based on population numbers) is devised to aggregate data by areal tracts. We have shown in this chapter various methods of analyzing disease data in areal representation, but the assumption of homogeneity of spatial units, as illustrated in the analysis of spatial autocorrelation, may not always be upheld.

Where point data fail to provide a continuous coverage or the patterns become confusing to interpret, areal-based analysis is essential to bring order and understanding to the spatial distribution of a variable of interest. Both point- and areal-based analytical approaches complement and supplement each other in describing a spatial pattern that may reveal an underlying process. We shall examine in the next chapter the correlation between disease incidents and sociodemographic characteristics in an attempt to enhance our understanding of the disease dynamics in relation to geographic location and other environmental artifacts.

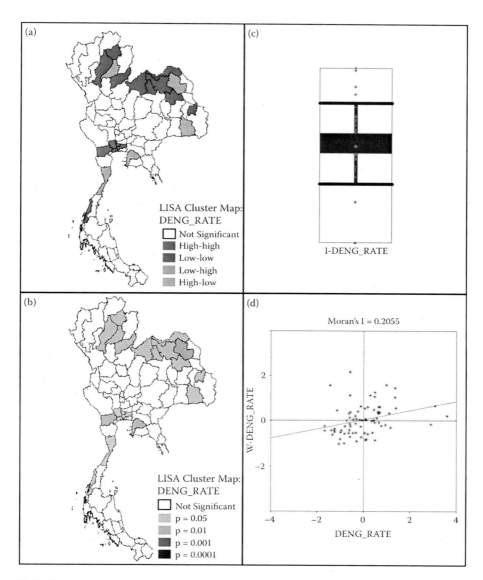

FIGURE 5.16
A color version of this figure follows page 108 Univariate LISA statistics in GeoDa.

References

1. Sherman, L.W., Hot spots of crime and criminal careers of places, in *Crime and Place*, Eck, J.E., and Weisburd, D., Eds., Criminal Justice Press, Monsey, NY, and Police Executive Research Forum, Washington, DC, 1995, 35.
2. Unwin, D., *Introductory Spatial Analysis*, Methuen, London, 1981, 212.

3. Evans, I.S., The selection of class intervals, *Transactions of the Institute of British Geographers*, 2, 98, 1977.
4. Holt, D., Steel, D.G., and Tranmer, M., Area homogeneity and the modifiable areal unit problem, *Geographical Systems*, 3, 181, 1996.
5. Moran, P.A.P., Notes on continuous stochastic phenomena, *Biometrika*, 37, 17, 1950.
6. Geary, R.C., The contiguity ratio and statistical mapping, *The Incorporated Statistician*, 5, 115, 1954.
7. Griffith, D.A., *Spatial Autocorrelation — A Primer*, Association of American Geographers, Washington, DC, 1987.
8. Anselin, L., *GeoDa 0.9 User's Guide, Spatial Analysis Laboratory*, Department of Agricultural and Consumer Economics and CSISS, University of Illinois, Urbana, IL, 2003. Available: http://www.sal.uiuc.edu/users/anselin/pdf/geoda_09.pdf [accessed on March 19, 2006].
9. Anselin, L., Local indicators of spatial association — LISA, *Geographical Analysis*, 27(2), 93, 1995.

6

Interpolation and Associative Analysis

6.1 Spatial Sampling and Interpolation

An interesting problem in spatial epidemiological study is largely attributable to the fact that most available data are in the form of complete enumeration of events based on administrative boundaries, such as census tracts within a fixed study area. Such data already form a realization and represent a completely mapped occurrence.[1] The problems of such a representation of aggregated data arising from zonation, as presented in Section 5.3.2 of Chapter 5, have sparked increased interest in spatial sampling that involves a limited number of locations in a geographic space to measure a phenomenon.

We have seen from Chapter 4 that the NNI is flawed because of its sensitivity toward the spatial scale of the study area. The method of quadrant counts uses grid cells of an arbitrarily defined size overlaid on the points. The number of points in each grid cell is counted and compared with the defined point of reference, that is, spatial randomness, via a χ^2 test of goodness of fit. Although this method is intuitive and easy to implement, the technique has a number of conceptual problems such as the arbitrariness in the choice of the grid cell size and the undermining of correlation between nearby cells. To solve this problem, a moving window approach called the kernel density estimation has emerged in point pattern analysis of disease data. In situations where a huge number of address data is available, particularly for data collected over long periods, the kernel density estimation approach can help the analysts simplify the complex point patterns without diminishing the significance of incident level data. The incident hot spots can then be verified and tested for their statistical significance against a random distribution.

Spatial sampling is a necessary procedure before spatial interpolation, but sampling methods in spatial epidemiology have not been fully developed over the years.[1] We reckon that data collected at sampled locations are representative of the spatial distribution. The interpolator will use these sample points to predict values of variables of interest at other unsampled locations. Numerous studies have shown that the method of sampling data points can have a great effect over the accuracy of the interpolation results. We use the asthma data set of Hong Kong to examine two scenarios: (1) kernel density, a realization method based on nearby events, and (2) interpolation, a spatial sampling approach. Both will generate statistical surfaces of varying degrees of smoothness.

6.1.1   Kernel Density Estimation

The kernel density estimation is a method for examining large-scale trends in point pattern analysis. It analyzes disease patterns and detects hot spots through a moving window technique linked to a quartic kernel algorithm. The approach attempts to estimate how event frequencies vary continuously across the study area based on the point patterns.[2,3] The kernel algorithm is implemented in some spatial analysis packages, including the geographic analysis machine,[4–6] spatial pattern analysis machine[7], and CrimeStat (demonstrated below), although parameters used in each of these packages differ slightly.

Figure 6.1 illustrates the kernel density approach in estimating event intensities from a number of points across a grid plate. The method involves a moving kernel represented by a three-dimensional function (k_i) of a defined radius or bandwidth (t_i) that visits every cell in the grid overlaid on the study area. When the kernel moves, distances are measured from either the intersections of the grids (g_i) or the centers of grid cells (gc_i) to each incident (s_i) falling within the bandwidth (t_i) (see Figure 6.1a and b). The simplest algorithm to estimate the intensity is by counting the number of disease incidents (s_i) detected within the circle to derive its intensity value. Alternatively, the quartic kernel estimation algorithm is used to calculate the intensity value for each point in the circle. The drawing of the many overlapping circles is repeated on each grid intersection (g_i) or grid center (gc_i) until the entire grid is covered. The closer an incident (s_i) is to a grid intersection (g_i) or grid center (gc_i), the higher the intensity value of that point. These intensity values are then summed up as the final intensity value of each circle.

Bandwidth in CrimeStat has a slightly different interpretation from the normal or the uniform kernel density modules. The defined bandwidth of the normal or uniform module is the standard deviation of the normal distribution. Instead, CrimeStat uses the radius of the search area for interpolation. The output of kernel estimation is usually a smooth continuous surface, such as a spatially based histogram. The degree at each location over the grid surface reflects the point pattern intensity of the neighboring areas.

Figures 6.2 and 6.3 illustrate the hot spots of asthma cases in Mongkok, a densely populated urban community in Kowloon, using the normal and

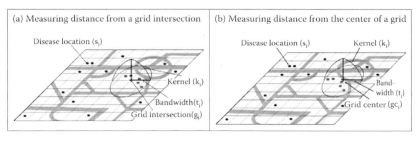

FIGURE 6.1
Kernel density estimation for point pattern analysis. (Adapted from Ratcliffe.[7])

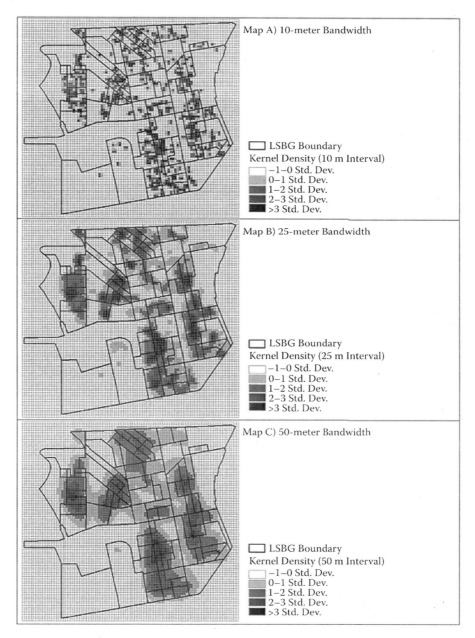

FIGURE 6.2
A comparison between changes of bandwidth intervals in normal kernel density interpolation using CrimeStat.

uniform kernel density interpolation methods, respectively, for three differ-ent bandwidths. Figure 6.2 uses the standard deviation of a normal distribu-tion as the defined bandwidth. With increasing bandwidths, the number of peaks on the resultant surfaces decreased and the degree of generalization maximized (maps A-C). A contour line can be drawn to delineate the extent and direction of the hot spots, which seem to extend vertically along Nathan Road in the middle right. The method offers intensity estimates over the entire study area.

Figure 6.3 shows the results of the uniform kernel density estimation of hot spots in which all points within the kernel were weighted equally. The only visually identifiable hot spot as evident in Figure 6.3 is situated in the lower middle portion of the study area (map F). Unlike the normal kernel, the uni-form kernel method estimates the intensity of a point within an area circum-scribed by the bandwidth, and the visual effect of its resultant maps are not as significant as those in Figure 6.2. Both sets of maps show that a smaller band-width increases the possibility of unidentifiable hot spots in the study area.

6.1.1.1   Kernel Density Estimation of Asthma Occurrences in Hong Kong

Objective:	To create a kernel density representation of asthma cases of Hong Kong
Software:	CrimeStat III
Epidemiological data:	Asthma data of Hong Kong, 1996–2000 (Table B.1 of Appendix B)
Boundary files:	Coastline and DC administrative boundaries of Hong Kong (Table B.6 of Appendix B)
Spatial scale:	Hong Kong

Step 1: Setting Up a Workspace in CrimeStat

Activate CrimeStat III as described in Step 1 of Section 4.3 of Chapter 4.

Step 2: Specifying Input Data

The procedure is as described in Step 2 of Section 4.3 but using the asthma data of Hong Kong (Table B.1 of Appendix B) as the input data.

Step 3: Specifying Grid Reference

Next, the extent and the grid size to superimpose on the study area must be defined for the kernel computation (Figure 6.4). The extent is controlled by coordinates of two opposite corners (usually the lower left and upper right) of a rectangular area that can be read into CrimeStat or keyed in manually. The

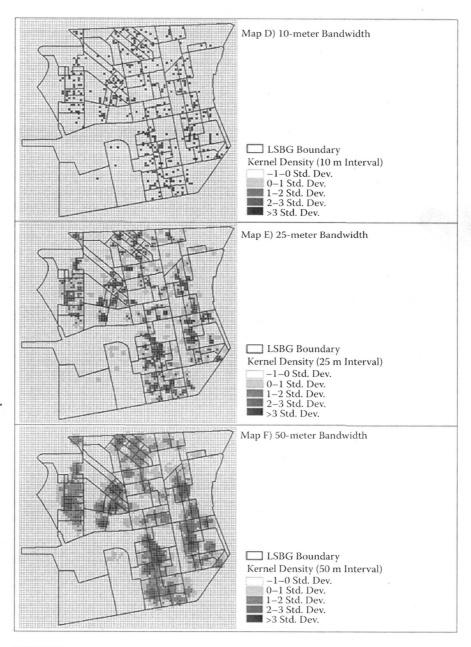

FIGURE 6.3
A comparison between changes of bandwidth intervals in uniform kernel density interpolation using CrimeStat.

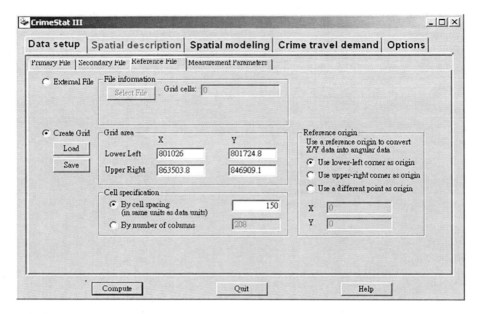

FIGURE 6.4
Specifying grid reference in CrimeStat.

specification must be in the same coordinate system and data units as in Step 2 earlier, although the latter may also be specified by "number of columns."

Step 4: Kernel Density Estimation

Kernel density estimation is an "Interpolation" function under "Spatial Modeling" in CrimeStat (Figure 6.5). Five methods of interpolation are available: (1) normal, (2) uniform, (3) quartic, (4) triangular, and (5) negative exponential.[2,8] The normal distribution method which extends to infinity in all directions is the most commonly used and suitable for disease modeling.[9] The method weighs all points in the study area with near points weighted more heavily than distant points.[10] The "Interval" or bandwidth should ideally be specified in the same data units in meters and not smaller than the grid size. A larger bandwidth will result in a smoother surface, but there is an increased possibility that hot spots may be concealed. The output or kernel density surface is stored in the shapefile format.

Step 5: Displaying Results of Kernel Density Estimation

CrimeStat is not equipped with map display functions. However, because the kernel density output from Step 4 above comes in the shapefile format, either GeoDa or HealthMapper can be used to display the results.

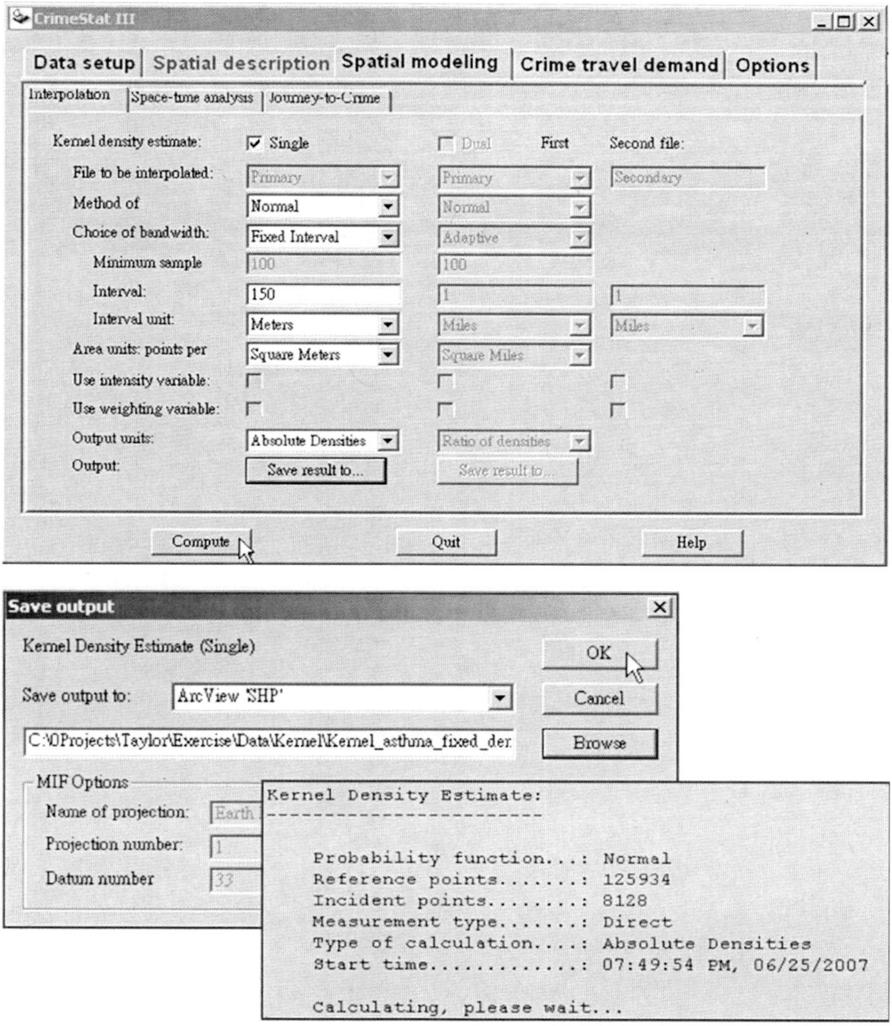

FIGURE 6.5
Kernel density estimation in CrimeStat.

Figure 6.6 shows two kernel density surfaces of asthma based on two different bandwidths that yield two very different looking maps. Map (a) exhibits a scattered pattern of hot spots of asthma, reflecting a close-to-reality pattern that mimics inhabited areas of Hong Kong. However, the spottiness makes the results difficult to handle. In contrast, map (b) reveals hot spots at about the same location, but its smoother appearance and continuous surface representation render it more readable. Figure 6.6 highlights the effects that bandwidth may have in kernel density estimation to be discussed in the next section.

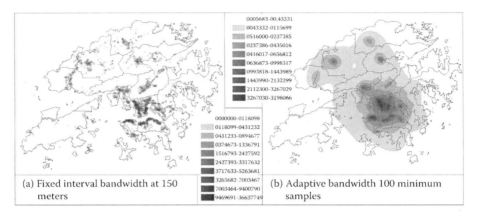

FIGURE 6.6
Kernel density surfaces based two different methods of bandwidths. Note: Kernel density was computed in CrimeStat, and results are displayed in HealthMapper.

6.1.1.2 Constraints and Limitations of the Kernel Density Method

6.1.1.2.1 Choice of a Bandwidth

The choice of a bandwidth is crucial in the kernel estimation because it determines the degree of smoothing applied on the point pattern. In general, a larger bandwidth yields a smoother surface with low intensity levels, whereas a smaller bandwidth produces a thorny surface with pronounced local variations. The choice of a bandwidth is research-specific, and there is no universal rule that would apply in every situation. Normally, the spatial extent and the intensity levels upon which to examine a phenomenon will determine the value of the bandwidth.

6.1.1.2.2 Choice of a Grid Size

Aside from bandwidth, grid size also affects the degree of smoothing on the kernel density estimation. Figure 6.7 shows two maps based on the uniform kernel estimation using two different grid sizes (a 50×50 m^2 grid in map A as opposed to a 100×100 m^2 grid in map B). A smaller grid cell covers a smaller area and naturally resembles more closely the pattern revealed in a point map. However, too small a grid cell defeats the aim of generalizing the point data into a smooth surface.

6.1.1.2.3 Census Tract versus Grid Cell Visualization

The choice of mapping methods and graphic variables conveying color, size, shape, and value are fundamental concerns in the process of mapmaking and design. The first step in a cartographic representation involves the selection of an aggregation level or the level of spatial discrimination to depict the data. Thus, a choice between using absolute representation (e.g., simple count) and relative representation (e.g., density) has to be made. A map based

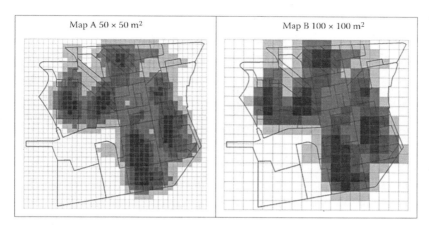

FIGURE 6.7
A comparison of two surfaces in different grid sizes based on normal kernel density interpolation. Note: Kernel density was computed in CrimeStat, and results are displayed in HealthMapper.

on simple counts can reveal a spatial distribution different from that based on density.[11]

The importance of selecting an appropriate areal unit in large-scale ecological studies on disease surveillance has been demonstrated in a body of literature. For example, the effects of socioeconomic factors were not apparent at the census tract level until subcensus tracts were examined.[12] Kamber et al.[13] advised that variation in block sizes would distort the analysis, thereby resulting in missed hot spots. Besides, the probability of missed hot spots occurred most likely in data covering a short period because too few data are available to differentiate between statistical noises. The usefulness of block-level analysis is thus constrained to small areas.

The most apparent merit of the grid cell method over the census tract method is the minimization of areal distortion imposed by fixed boundaries. The fact that transport arteries are used to delimit census tracts creates problems in presenting the data. For example, it is common to find disease hot spots across tracts rather than confined within predefined administrative boundaries. Modelers usually prefer the use of grids in time-series analysis of hot spot identification because administrative boundaries are unavoidably subject to change for political reasons and do not favor comparison of disease patterns over consecutive periods (e.g., month-by-month or week-by-week comparisons in successive years).

6.1.2 Spatial Interpolation Methods

Interpolation predicts unknown values for cells in a raster format using data from a limited number of sample geographic points. Its basic assumption is that spatially distributed objects are correlated and things that are closer tend to have similar values. Some applications of spatial interpolation include the modeling of surfaces based on readings of temperature or soil pH. An interpolated surface can be a complete statistical surface, a contour map, a triangulated irregular network (TIN) file, or a raster file with estimated point values.

The three commonly used spatial interpolation methods in a GIS include the following: (1) Inverse Distance Weighted (IDW), (2) spline, and (3) kriging. IDW and spline are regarded as the deterministic approach because they are directly based on nearby measured values or mathematical formulae. Kriging, on the other hand, is based on spatial statistics, and the weighting of each sample point is worked out by a matrix.

6.1.2.1   *IDW and Its Constraints*

IDW is also called the moving average or distance weighted average method. It assumes that each sample point has a local influence that diminishes with distance such that the closer a point is to the center of the cell being estimated, the more influence or weight it has in the averaging process. There are almost infinite varieties of IDW algorithms, including variations by nature of the distance function, number of observed points, and direction in choosing sample points.

IDW is the most widely used method and the easiest to handle in spatial interpolation. The resultant surface tends to be smooth, as can be seen from a surface of air pollution (Figure 6.8). However, the method has a few pitfalls: (1) the range of interpolated values is limited by the range of the data and (2) the number of sampling points and their locations are crucial to the outcome. Because no interpolated value will be outside the range of observed values, peaks and pits will be overlooked if they are not sampled. The characteristics of the interpolated layer will be less accurate were sampling points not distributed in a proper way.

IDW interpolation has two operating parameters needing particular attention: power and radius. In general, a higher power means more emphasis will be put on nearer points, thus resulting in a rigid-looking surface. Radius is used to determine the number of known points to estimate an unknown value. A fixed radius is chosen when known points are plentiful and are regularly distributed over a study area. A variable radius is preferred when sample points are sparsely distributed. The efficiency of the interpolation is also subject to the number of sampled points included in the averaging and the regularity of the sampled points.

6.1.2.2   *Spline and Its Constraints*

Spline estimates values by using a mathematical function to minimize the overall surface curvature to yield a smooth surface that passes through the input points.[14] Because this method minimizes the total curvature to result in a relatively smooth surface, spline is usually adopted in modeling gently varying surfaces such as elevation, water table heights, or population concentrations.

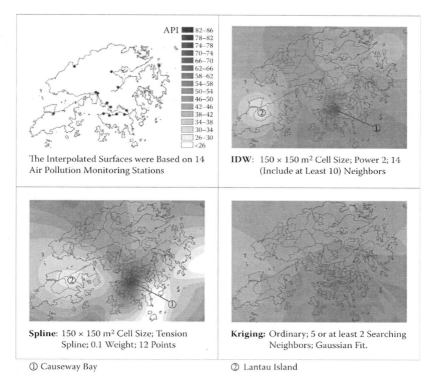

The Interpolated Surfaces were Based on 14 Air Pollution Monitoring Stations	**IDW:** 150 × 150 m^2 Cell Size; Power 2; 14 (Include at Least 10) Neighbors
Spline: 150 × 150 m^2 Cell Size; Tension Spline; 0.1 Weight; 12 Points	**Kriging:** Ordinary; 5 or at least 2 Searching Neighbors; Gaussian Fit.

① Causeway Bay ② Lantau Island

FIGURE 6.8
Surfaces of API of Hong Kong using three interpolation methods. Note: Interpolation was done in Geostatistical Analyst and Spatial Analyst.

The advantage of spline is also its inherent problem. Although this method allows for the choice of number of points used in an interpolation, many of the cells may need to be reduced to fit in a certain surface with as small a curvature as possibly achievable. The maximum number of bends in a splined surface is limited to 10 because the output is possibly not readable if the limit is exceeded. Therefore, spline is not suitable for modeling a phenomenon with a substantial range of values in certain parts of the study area.

6.1.2.3 Kriging (Ordinary or Universal) and Its Constraints

Kriging is a geostatistical interpolation method introduced by Matheron[15] as the "theory of regionalized variables" and by Krige[16] as an optimal interpolation method for use in the mining industry. Although similar to the IDW in the assignment of differential weights to known points in the estimation of unknown values, the weights assigned are not based solely on distance measures but also on the spatial autocorrelation factor. A key characteristic of kriging is its ability to model irregular variations over a surface.[17] For instance, a cohort of population is found more susceptible to certain types of illnesses, and this observation is expected to affect the regularity of weights assigned to the interpolation process.

Kriging concerns the rate at which the variance between points changes over space. This is expressed through a semivariogram (see Explanation Box 6.1), which shows how the average difference between values at points changes with distance between points. Because the absolute value of a point can only be estimated, a semivariogram is used to provide measures of sample variability, range of influence, and sample adequacy. Simple kriging assumes that the surface has a constant mean and has no underlying trend and that all variation is statistical. Universal kriging assumes that there is a deterministic trend in the surface that underlies the statistical variation. In either case, once trends have been accounted for (or assumed not to exist), all other variation is assumed to be a function of distance.

Kriging is a rather complicated method in attaining a statistical surface and may require intensive computer resources when the number of sample points is large. The complexity in operating and defining kriging parameters is much higher than in the other two methods. A slight difference of one parameter could result in a completely different surface. The accuracy of the interpolated surface is very much dependent on the experience of the analyst, and there is no universal rule that can suit all applications.

6.1.2.4   *Spatial Interpolation of Air Pollution Index (API) of Hong Kong*

Freeware for doing spatial interpolation operations is not easy to find because the procedures are more algorithmic-intensive. Most interpolation software requires an official and paid registration after an evaluation period. The Integrated Land and Water Information System (ILWIS) is a rare freeware for interpolation. It was developed by the International Institute for Aerospace Survey and Earth Sciences in the Netherlands and is available for download at www.itc.nl/ilwis/. There are many functions available in ILWIS, including data conversion between vector and raster formats, image processing tools, and geostatistical analyses with kriging for interpolation. Unfortunately, we found the export functions for TXT and SHP unstable; hence, its use is not covered in this book.

Figure 6.8 was prepared using the Geostatistical Analyst extension on air pollution data of Hong Kong to exemplify differences among the three interpolation techniques discussed above (IDW, spline, and kriging).[18] It can be seen that different interpolators will produce different models, and there is no hard and fast rule about which method best represents a continuous phenomenon. The IDW surface is able to capture the peaks and pits across the land area but not in the water areas without any sample point. The spline surface is comparatively smoother than that of IDW, but again, the water and peripheral areas with no sample points affect the accuracy of the interpolation. Both IDW and spline surfaces correctly indicate two widely known facts about Hong Kong: (1) the Causeway Bay area has the worst air quality and (2) Lantau Island has the best air quality. Our Gaussian model (and, in fact,

Explanation Box 6.1: Computing and interpreting a semivariogram.
A semivariogram is a graphic display of semivariance (γ) versus distance or lag (see diagram below). Semivariance is a measure of the degree of spatial dependence or autocorrelation between samples. To compute a semivariogram, we need to determine how variance behaves against distance. First, we divide the range of distance into a set of discrete intervals, for example, 10 intervals between zero and maximum distance in the study area. Then, we compute distance and the squared difference in z values for every pair of points. Each pair of points is assigned to one of the distance ranges and the total variance in each range is accumulated. When every pair has been used (or a sample of pairs in a large data set), the average variance in each distance range is computed. We can plot this value at the midpoint distance of each range and fit one of a standard set of curves (e.g., spherical, cubic, exponential, Gaussian, linear) to the points. The choice of theoretical model is determined largely by experience and experimentation.

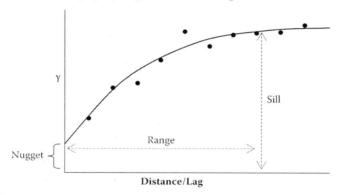

At a certain distance, the model levels out. The distance where the model first flattens out is known as the range and the corresponding value on the y axis is called the sill. Samples separated by distances closer than the range are spatially autocorrelated, whereas locations farther apart than the range are not. The range is thus the distance beyond which the deviation in z values does not depend on distance. The intersection of the model with the y axis is called the nugget, where a nonzero nugget indicates that repeated measurements at the same point yield different values in developing the semivariogram. Once the semivariogram has been developed, it is used to estimate distance weights for interpolation.

all models) by the ordinary kriging method does not seem to yield a realistic surface, primarily because of insufficient sample points. Moreover, the 14 monitoring stations are not evenly distributed throughout Hong Kong, and there is little representation toward the outer extent of the territory.

Figure 6.8 also shows that interpolation must be handled with care for areas that are not continuous, such as the case of Hong Kong and many countries in Asia. This deficiency could be overcome by considering the shorelines as breaklines in some software. A comparison of some characteristics of the three methods is shown in Table 6.1.

6.2   Associate Analysis

We have seen in Chapter 4 (Figure 4.14) that several SARS clusters were identified by using the SDEs, but they provided no explanation for the phenomenon. Similarly, hot spots of asthma as revealed in Figures 6.2 and 6.3 cannot be explained without further investigation. Disease mapping has a long history in spatial epidemiological studies and has been used specifically for visualization of diseases and hypothesis generation.[19] Jacquez[20] and

TABLE 6.1

A Comparison of Characteristics of Three Interpolation Methods

	IDW	Spline	Kriging
Assumption	Deterministic; changes in the parts near the sampling points would be more intense than the parts farther from it	Deterministic; based directly on measured values nearby and mathematical formulae	Spatial statistics; the weights assigned are not based solely on distance measures but also on the spatial autocorrelation factor
Best for	Variable being mapped decreases in influence with distance from the sampled locations	Gradually varying surfaces	When there is a spatially correlated distance or directional bias in the data
Example	Ozone concentration	Elevation, water table heights, and pollution concentration	Soil science and geology
Inherited disadvantage	Range of interpolated values is limited by the range of the data	Not suitable to model phenomenon with extreme values	Complexity in operating and defining kriging parameters
	Number of sampling points and their locations affect outcome	Not appropriate when there are large changes within a short horizontal distance	Accuracy of the interpolated surface depended on the experience of analyst

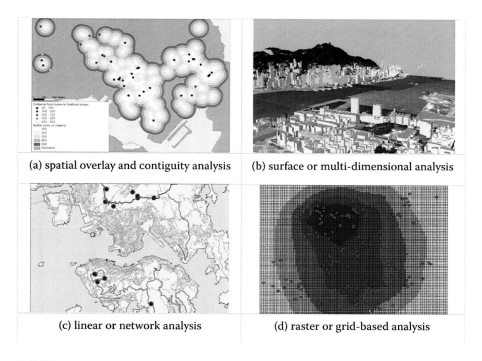

(a) spatial overlay and contiguity analysis

(b) surface or multi-dimensional analysis

(c) linear or network analysis

(d) raster or grid-based analysis

FIGURE 1.10
Types of spatial data analysis: (a) spatial overlay and contiguity analysis, (b) surface or multidimensional analysis, (c) linear or network analysis, and (d) raster- or grid-based analysis.

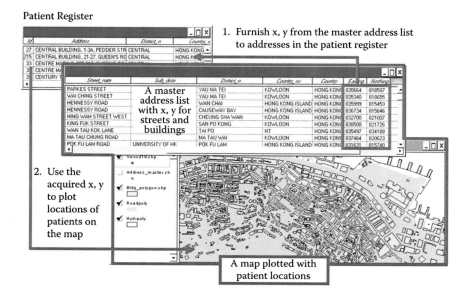

FIGURE 2.6
Address matching or geocoding.

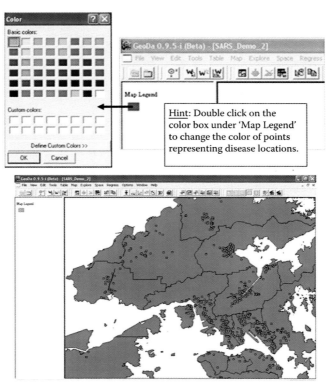

FIGURE 4.4
Changing symbol color in GeoDa.

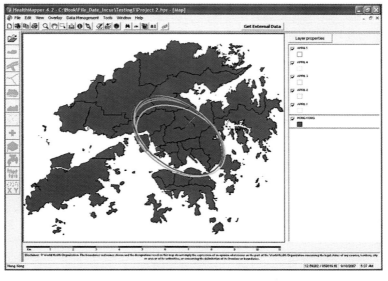

FIGURE 4.12
Displaying results of SDE in the HealthMapper.

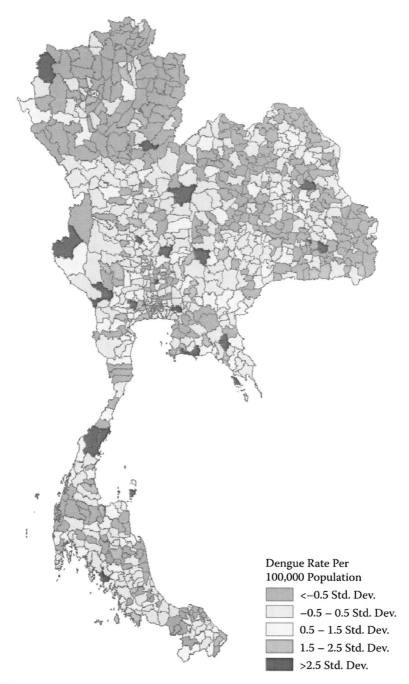

**Dengue Rate Per
100,000 Population**

▢ <−0.5 Std. Dev.
▢ −0.5 − 0.5 Std. Dev.
▢ 0.5 − 1.5 Std. Dev.
▢ 1.5 − 2.5 Std. Dev.
▢ >2.5 Std. Dev.

FIGURE 5.3
A map of dengue rate by province in Thailand using the standard deviation method in
GeoDa.

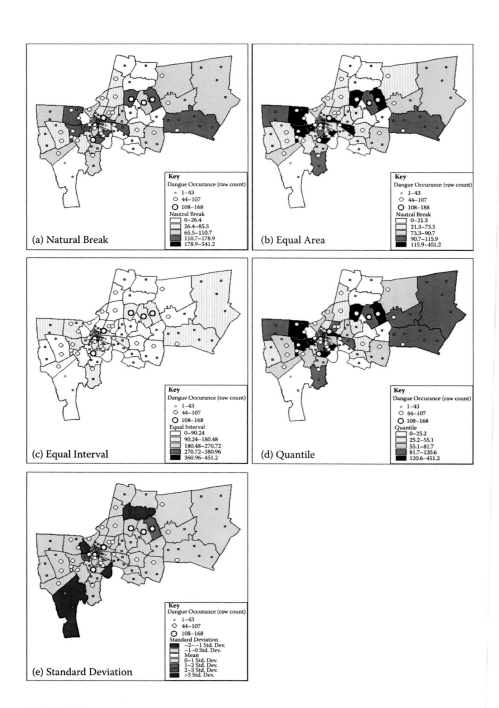

FIGURE 5.7
Maps of dengue rates per 100,000 population in Bangkok using different classification methods.

For each location, LISA values allow for the computation of its similarity with its neighbors and also to test its significance. Five scenarios may emerge:

■	High-high	**Hot spots** or locations with high values with similar neighbors
■	Low-low	**Cold spots** or locations with low values with similar neighbors
■	Low-high	Potential **spatial outliers** or locations with low values with high-value neighbors
■	High-low	Potential **spatial outliers** or locations with high values with low-value neighbors
□	Not Significant	Locations with **no significant local autocorrelation**

FIGURE 5.10
Local indicators of spatial association.

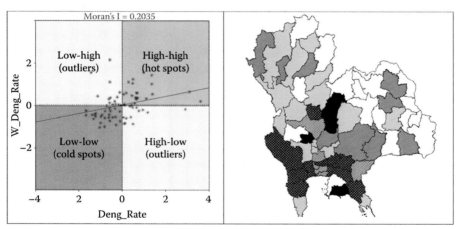

Note: Highlighting the first quadrant on the scatter plot (left) reveals provinces belonging to the 'High-high' (hot spots) category (right)

FIGURE 5.14
A Moran scatterplot in GeoDa.

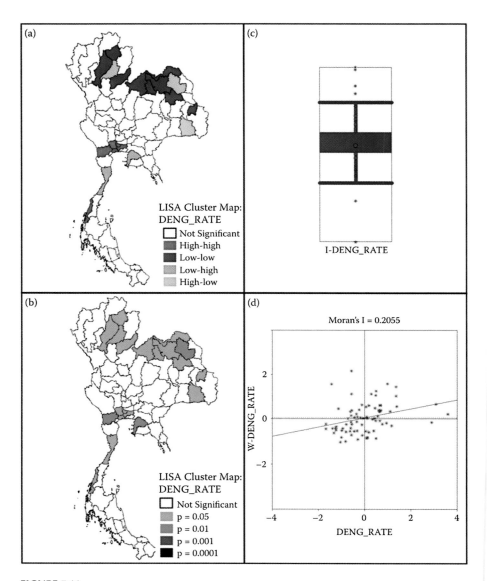

FIGURE 5.16
Univariate LISA statistics in GeoDa.

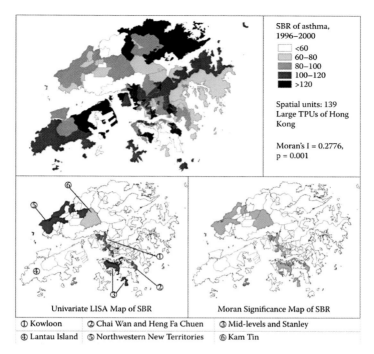

FIGURE 6.9
SBR of asthma by large TPUs of Hong Kong. Note: Univariate LISA and Moran significance map were done in GeoDa.

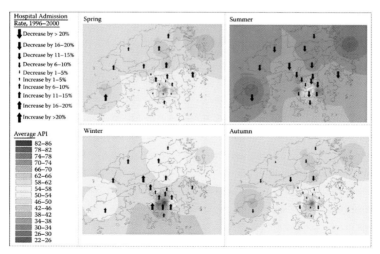

FIGURE 6.11
Spatial overlay of hospital admission rate of asthma against seasonal variation of average API of Hong Kong, 1996–2000. Note: Seasonal variations of asthma admissions are indicated as rates above or below the overall average admission rate of Hong Kong. Interpolation method: IDW, 150 × 150 m² cell size; power, 2; 14 (include at least 10) neighbors. Software: Geostatistical Analyst. (Data from Hospital Authority and Environmental Protection Department of Hong Kong.)

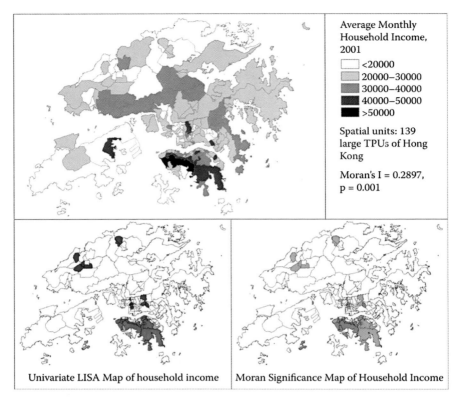

Average Monthly Household Income, 2001

☐ <20000
20000–30000
30000–40000
40000–50000
■ >50000

Spatial units: 139 large TPUs of Hong Kong

Moran's I = 0.2897, p = 0.001

Univariate LISA Map of household income | Moran Significance Map of Household Income

FIGURE 6.12
Average monthly household income by large TPUs of Hong Kong. Note: Univariate LISA and Moran significance map were done in GeoDa.

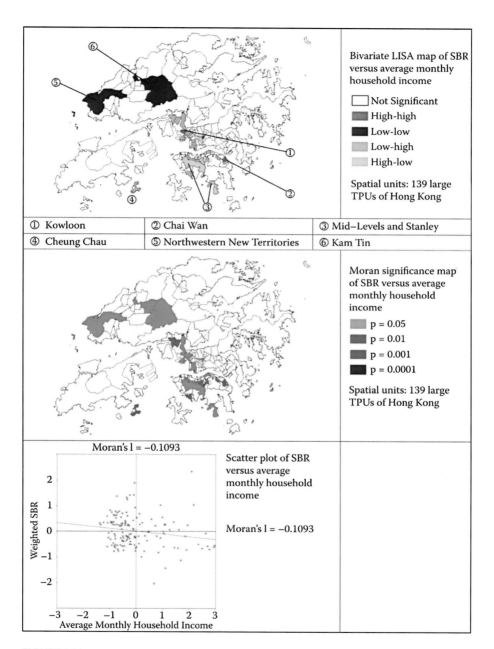

FIGURE 6.14
Spatial autocorrelation between SBR of asthma and average monthly household income by large TPU of Hong Kong. Note: Bivariate LISA and Moran significance map were done in GeoDa.

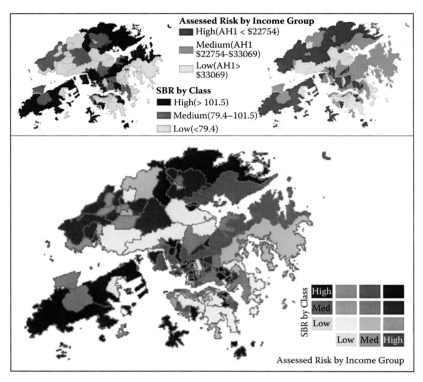

FIGURE 6.15
A bivariate map of SBR and average monthly household income (AHI) by large TPU of Hong Kong using ArcGIS.

Yu et al.[21] argued that GIS not only is a system designed for making disease maps but also leads to a better understanding of the causative relationships between the environment and human health. Evan and Stoddart[22] recognized three determinants of health: (1) genetic, (2) socioeconomic, and (3) biophysical. The above observations suggested explanations through sociodemographic variables, physical premises, or nearby land use and environmental characteristics.

For the remainder of this chapter, we will demonstrate how data on asthma admissions in Hong Kong can be associated with environmental and socioeconomic factors. We select API as the environmental factor and average monthly household income by large TPU as the socioeconomic factor. The examples make use of the Standardized Morbidity Ratio (SBR; refer to Section 3.4.1 of Chapter 3 for the formula to compute the SMR) of asthma against other factors using the spatial overlay techniques available in most GIS. Put simply, the SBR is a ratio of the observed number of hospital admissions (not necessarily mortality in the numerator as implied in the SMR) to the expected number multiplied by 100. An SBR value of less than 100 implies that the morbidity rate is lower than that for Hong Kong as a whole, and vice versa. The spatial overlay technique[23] in spatial epidemiology often involves superimposing a map of disease incidence over another map of a variable suspected to have a possible association (e.g., SBR of asthma and air pollution, SBR of asthma and household income). The former involves the combined use of a surface of disease incidence against an interpolated (continuous) surface, whereas the latter combines a surface of disease incidence against a census enumeration (partitioned) surface.

Figure 6.9 shows a map of SBR of asthma by 139 large TPUs of Hong Kong (after consolidating TPUs of very small areas of the same constituencies into larger spatial units). The spatial pattern exhibits some degree of clustering (Moran's $I = 0.2776$, $p = .001$) with hot spots in Kowloon and Chai Wan (northeast of the Hong Kong Island). These areas correspond to communities with light industries. The cold spots are found in the more affluent regions of Mid-Levels and Stanley of the Hong Kong Island, as well as the sparsely populated and horticultural regions to the northwest of New Territories. There are also pockets of outliers in which these areas register SBR values dissimilar from (i.e., much higher or lower than) the average rates of their neighbors.

6.2.1 Application of Interpolated Surface in Associate Analysis: The Risk of Asthma Relative to API of Hong Kong

Environment and health are closely related and environmental influence on health has been studied in medical science.[24] The adverse effects of air pollution are well documented and experimented in medical research and surveys, as well as from the geographic perspective. Studies have concentrated on such topics as disease clustering, cluster identification, association with point sources of pollution, and space–time disease incidence.[25,26] The space–time clustering of disease is defined by incidence rates that are higher in

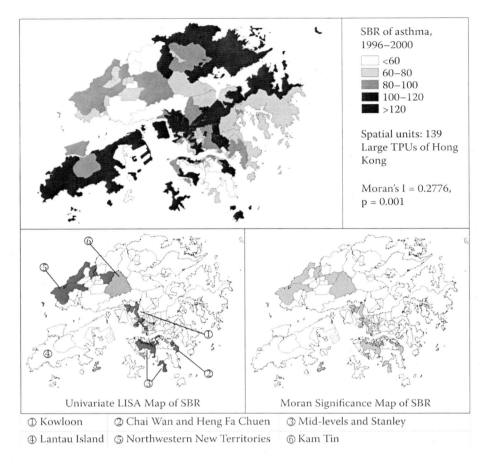

① Kowloon	② Chai Wan and Heng Fa Chuen	③ Mid-levels and Stanley
④ Lantau Island	⑤ Northwestern New Territories	⑥ Kam Tin

FIGURE 6.9
A color version of this figure follows page 108 SBR of asthma by large TPUs of Hong Kong.
Note: Univariate LISA and Moran significance map were done in GeoDa.

some places than in others and higher at some periods than at others.[27] These studies included tests to determine the significance of clustering because the observed disease incidence could have arisen by chance alone, confounded by unknown variables or by known covariates.[28]

Temporal influence over disease occurrences is significant because people's activity space changes with time. For example, the residents of Hong Kong are more susceptible to respiratory illnesses (e.g., asthma in Figure 6.9) beginning in the month of September and through the winter months partly because of seasonal factors but also because more people have returned to work or school, resulting in close contact of high intensity in daily commuting. Figure 6.10 shows that APIs in the summer months (June–August) are comparatively lower than those during the winter months (December–February).

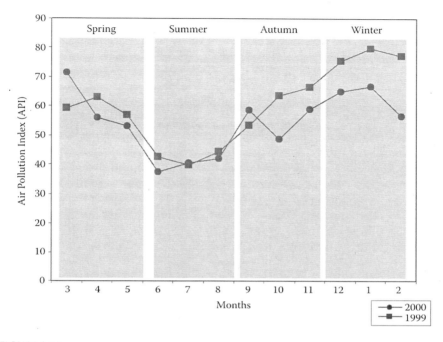

FIGURE 6.10

Monthly API in Hong Kong, 1999–2000 (spring, March–May; summer, June–August; autumn, September–November; winter, December–February). (Data from Environmental Protection Department.[32])

Plenty of medical research in Hong Kong has shown a positive relationship between air pollution and mortality in respiratory diseases, including asthma.[29–31] This section cartographically and statistically examines the spatial autocorrelation between air pollution and asthma. A total of 14 air quality monitoring sites in Hong Kong (Figure 6.8a) have been recording air pollutant concentration on a daily basis since 1999.[32] Figure 6.11 shows the seasonal variation of air pollution in Hong Kong as reflected by the average API.

The brownish shadings (see color insert) found in autumn, winter, and spring (top left and bottom row in Figure 6.11) reflect higher API values recorded during these months. The highest APIs were recorded in the central and western districts of the Hong Kong Island and in the southern part of the Kowloon peninsula. The greenish shadings indicate relatively better API readings or air quality in the summer months (top right in Figure 6.11). It can be seen from Figure 6.11 that asthma admissions were higher than the overall average for winter when the air quality was poor. Although admissions of asthma cases also exceeded the average level in spring, the intensity was less severe. Conversely, the summer months recorded below-average admissions of asthma cases. Further analysis by statistical means between air quality and asthma admissions was not attempted because the two layers were not of the same spatial units or measurement scales.

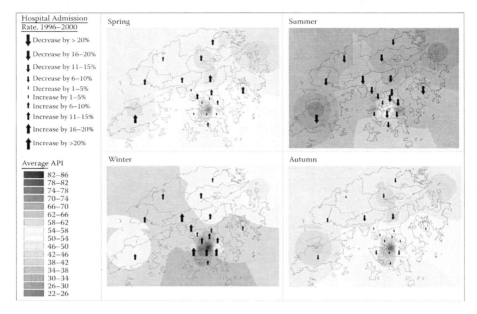

FIGURE 6.11

A color version of this figure follows page 108 Spatial overlay of hospital admission rate of asthma against seasonal variation of average API of Hong Kong, 1996–2000. Note: Seasonal variations of asthma admissions are indicated as rates above or below the overall average admission rate of Hong Kong. Interpolation method: IDW, 150 × 150 m² cell size; power, 2; 14 (include at least 10) neighbors. Software: Geostatistical Analyst. (Data from Hospital Authority and Environmental Protection Department of Hong Kong.)

6.2.2 Application of Socioeconomic Data in Associate Analysis: Risk of Asthma Relative to Monthly Household Income of the Population of Hong Kong

The significance of socioeconomic factors to health has been one of the major research themes in medical studies.[21,33–35] Socioeconomic variables have always been used to measure and explain disease patterns because social class is believed to demonstrate a close association with health behaviors. The cross-comparison of disease distribution against other spatial units is an imperative process. Such comparisons would allow a researcher to hypothesize a situation with more focus and explore possible relationships between the selected socioeconomic variables and disease incidence.

Socioeconomic analysis provides an understanding of the demographic and physical differences between high- and low-disease enumeration units. Lloyd et al.[33] characterized diseases based on wealth as either affluent or deprived. Figure 6.12 shows the spatial pattern by average monthly household income of Hong Kong in 2001. It is clear that higher-income groups, such as those with a monthly household income of more than HK$50,000, are concentrated in the middle and southern parts of the Hong Kong Island (Moran's *I* value = 0.2897, *p* = .001). Households with lower income were more

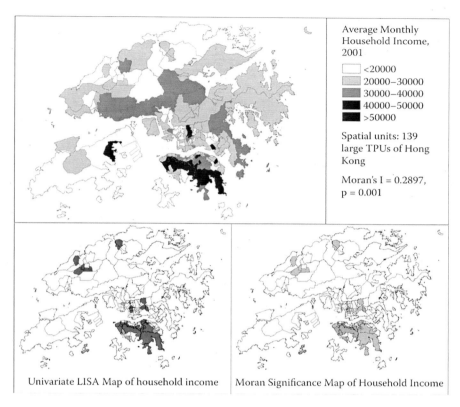

FIGURE 6.12

A color version of this figure follows page 108 Average monthly household income by large TPUs of Hong Kong. Note: Univariate LISA and Moran significance map were done in GeoDa.

widespread in the western and northern portions of the New Territories, Lantau, and pockets of areas in Kowloon.

Figure 6.13 shows the Pearson correlation between the SBR of asthma and various groups in terms of average monthly household income based on 139 large TPUs. The correlation coefficients also show SBRs to exhibit a significant negative relationship with the top two income groups but a significant positive relationship with the remaining groups except the lowest-income group (those earning less than HK$1,999). Although the income factor may not directly imply asthma, it has been observed that people with lower income are prone to accept higher health risks from occupational and environmental exposures.[36] Therefore, the confirmation of the income factor not only helps develop the policy for health care planning but also forms the target for environmental education programs.

When this income map is correlated with the SBRs of asthma in Hong Kong (Figure 6.14), it is apparent that low SBRs are found mostly with high-

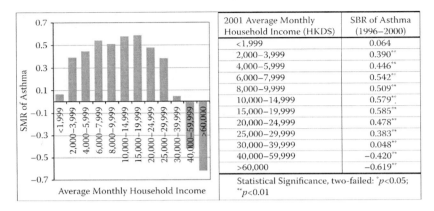

2001 Average Monthly Household Income (HKDS)	SBR of Asthma (1996–2000)
<1,999	0.064
2,000–3,999	0.390**
4,000–5,999	0.446**
6,000–7,999	0.542**
8,000–9,999	0.509**
10,000–14,999	0.579**
15,000–19,999	0.585**
20,000–24,999	0.478**
25,000–29,999	0.383**
30,000–39,999	0.048**
40,000–59,999	−0.420**
>60,000	−0.619**
Statistical Significance, two-failed: *$p<0.05$; **$p<0.01$	

FIGURE 6.13
Correlation between SBR of asthma and average monthly household income of Hong Kong. (Data from Hospital Authority and Census and Statistics Department of Hong Kong.)

income areas of Mid-Levels and Stanley (the high–low spatial outliers). In contrast, high SBRs are associated with the lower-income areas mostly situated in Kowloon (the low-high spatial outliers). The hot spots of high-high positive autocorrelation of reasonably high income and high disease rate are Mei Foo in Kowloon and Heng Fa Chuen in Hong Kong Island. The cold spots of low-low positive autocorrelation are again in the agricultural and sparsely population suburbs of northwest New Territory.

Another way of representing a map overlay of two layers is by means of the bivariate choropleth mapping technique (Figure 6.15).[37] Two related variables are each classed into not more than three categories representing low, medium, and high values and then mapped against each other. The result is a map comprising nine shades (the larger map in Figure 6.15) to indicate association between the two variables. We can see from the map legend that the diagonal shadings (going from bottom left to upper right) indicate positive correlations (high–high, medium–medium, and low–low), and the remaining shadings show some discrepancies. Such a map display is difficult for new users to interpret, and nine shadings is probably the limit for most readers. Besides using the same enumeration units, the effectiveness of the display is dependent on how the two original variables are classed.

Figures 6.14 and 6.15 are attempts to display the spatial association of two variables. The former draws on neighborhood similarities, whereas the latter shows a direct comparison at the same location. The patterns displayed have little similarities, although the same data sets are used. The difference arises primarily from data classification of the choropleth maps in Figure 6.15, as discussed in Section 5.3.1 of Chapter 5.

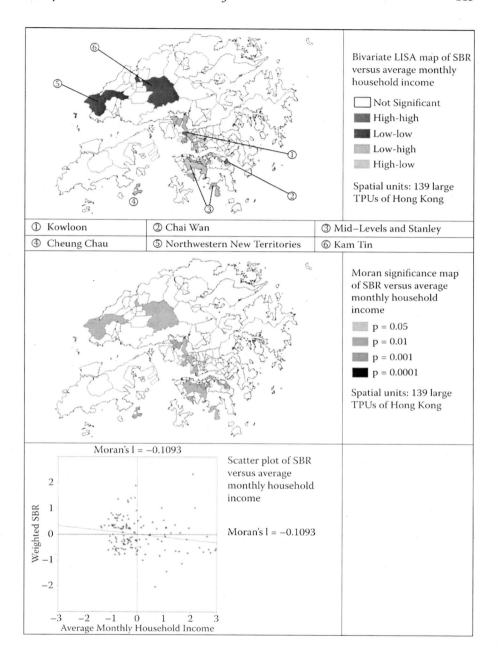

FIGURE 6.14

A color version of this figure follows page 108 Spatial autocorrelation between SBR of asthma and average monthly household income by large TPU of Hong Kong. Note: Bivariate LISA and Moran significance map were done in GeoDa.

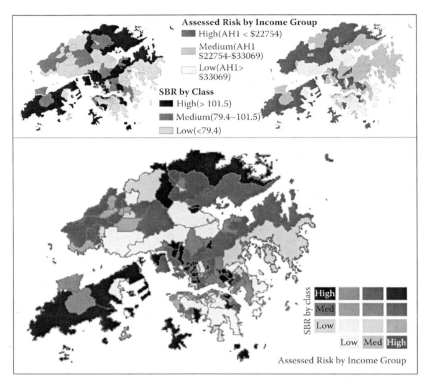

FIGURE 6.15
A color version of this figure follows page 108 A bivariate map of SBR and average monthly household income (AHI) by large TPU of Hong Kong using ArcGIS.

6.3 Summary

Different types of cartographic and geostatistical analyses have been used in this chapter. Although the kernel density estimation approach offers a number of practical advantages over the use of census tracts in visualizing complex disease patterns, it is not suitable for analyzing socioeconomic association. Aggregation of data by census tracts can be a useful method of data collation for data in different levels of resolution (e.g., individuals, households, establishments such as schools and businesses) because all objects can be brought to a common spatial ground.

Our analysis suggests that using population-level hospitalization data and a broad range of spatial analytical methods helps address the following objectives: (1) to examine seasonal variation in asthma hospitalization, (2) to investigate the existence of spatial variation of asthma hospitalization at the district and TPU levels, and (3) to understand the role of social and environmental characteristics in determining spatial variation. Our examples showed the presence of significant spatial clusters of hospitalization rates of asthma in Kowloon and Chai Wan. Our cartographic analysis revealed a direct association between air pollution and asthma in Hong Kong. A negative relationship between income and asthma was also observed. The notion of a respiratory illness, or asthma in this case, as a "disease of deprivation" is further confirmed.

The next chapter will offer guidelines on the adoption of a GIS approach in spatial epidemiological studies and disease analyses.

References

1. Lawson, A.B., Statistical *Methods in Spatial Epidemiology*, Wiley, Chichester, 2001.
2. Bailey, T., and Gatrell, A., *Interactive Spatial data Analysis*, Wiley, New York, NY, 1995.
3. Williamson, D., McLafferty, S., Goldsmith, V., McGuire, P., and Mollenkopf, J., Smoothing crime incident data: new methods for determining the bandwidth in kernel estimation, in *Proceedings ESRI User Conference*, San Diego, CA, July 27–31, 1998. Available: http://gis.esri.com/library/userconf/proc98/PROCEED/TO850/PAP829/P829.HTM [Accessed on October 15, 2007].
4. Openshaw, S., and Mark, A., Geographical analysis machine for the automated analysis of point data sets, *International Journal of Geographical Information Science*, 1, 4, 335–358, 1987.
5. Openshaw, S., Craft, A.W., Charlton, M., and Birch, J.M., Investigation of leukemia clusters by use of geographical analysis machine, *Lancet*, 1, 272, 1988.
6. Openshaw, S., Turton, I., and Macgill, J., Using the geographical analysis machine to analyze limiting long-term illness census data, *Geographical & Environmental Modelling*, 3(1), 83, 1999.
7. Ratcliffe, J., *Spatial Pattern Analysis Machine*, n.d. Available: http://jratcliffe.net/ware/spam1.htm [Accessed on October 15, 2007].
8. Burt, J.E., and Barber, G., *Elementary Statistics for Geographers*, Guilford Press, London, 1996.
9. Kelsall, J.E., and Diggle, P.J., Non-parametric estimation of spatial variation in relative risk, *Statistics in Medicine*, 14, 2335, 1995.
10. Levine, N., *CrimeStat: A Spatial Statistics Program for the Analysis of Crime Incident Locations*, Version 3.1, Ned Levine & Associates, Houston, TX, and the National Institute of Justice, Washington, DC, March 2007.
11. Kraak, M., and Ormeling, F., *Cartography: Visualization of Spatial Data*, Longman, Essex, 1996.
12. Cohen, J., Blumstein, A., and Miller, H., Demographically disaggregated projections of prison populations, Journal of Criminal Justice, 8(1), 1, 1980.
13. Kamber, T., Mollenkopf, J.H., and Ross, T.A., Crime, space and place: an analysis of crime patterns in Brooklyn, in *Analysing Crime Patterns: Frontiers of Practice*, Goldsmith, V., McGuire, P., Mollenkopf, J., and Ross, T.A., Eds., Sage Publications, London, 2000, 107.

14. Schoenberg, I.J., Contributions to the problem of approximation of equidistant data by analytic functions, *Quarterly of Applied Mathematics*, 4, 45, 1946.

15. Matheron, G., Principles of geostatistics, *Economic Geology*, 58, 1246, 1963.

16. Krige, D.G., *A Statistical Approach to Some Mine Valuations and Allied Problems at the Witwatersrand*, Master's thesis, University of Witwatersrand, Johannesburg, 1951.

17. Croner, C.M., and De Cola, L., Visualization of Disease Surveillance Data With Geostatistics, UNECE *Work Session on Methodological Issues Involving Integration of Statistics and Geography*, Tallinn, September 25–28, 2001. Available: http://www.unece.org/stats/documents/2001/09/gis/25.e.pdf [Accessed on October 15, 2007].

18. Johnston, K.M., Ver Hoef, M., Krivoruchko, K., and Lucas, N., *Using the Geostatistical Analyst*, ESRI Press, CA, 2001.

19. Cliff, A.D., and Haggett, P., *Atlas of Disease Distributions: Analytic Approaches to Epidemiological Data*, Blackwell, Oxford, 1988.

20. Jacquez, G.M., GIS as an enabling technology, in *GIS and Health*, Gatrell, A.G., and Loytonen, M., Eds., Taylor & Francis, London, 1988, Chap. 2.

21. Yu, T.S., Wong, S.L., Wong, T.W., and Lloyd, O.L., Mortality mapping in Hong Kong, 1979–83 and 1984–88: the patterns of major non-malignant diseases, *Asia Pacific Public Health*, 8(2), 74, 1995.

22. Evans, R.G., and Stoddart, G.L., Producing health, consuming health care, *Social Science and Medicine*, 31, 1347, 1990.

23. Tomlin, D., *Geographic Information Systems and Cartographic Modeling*, Prentice-Hall, Englewood Cliffs, NJ, 1990.

24. Rowland, A.J., and Cooper, P., *Environment and Health*, Edward Arnold Publishers, London, 1983.

25. Marshall, R.J., Mapping disease and mortality rates using empirical Bayes estimators, *Applied Statistics*, 40, 283, 1991.

26. Elliot, P., Wakefield, J.C., Best, N., and Briggs, D., *Spatial Epidemiology: Methods and Applications*, Oxford University Press, Oxford, 2000.

27. Rothman, K., A sobering start to the cluster-busters conference, *American Journal of Epidemiology*, 132, S6–S12, 1990.

28. Ripley, B.D., Modelling spatial patterns [with discussion], *Journal of Royal Statistical Society* B, 39, 172, 1977.

29. Chan-Yeung, M., Air pollution and health, *Hong Kong Medical Journal*, 6, 390, 2000.

30. Wong, C.M., Ma, S., Hedley, A.J., and Lam, T.H., Effect of air pollution in daily mortality in Hong Kong, *Environmental Health Perspectives*, 109(4), 335, 2001.

31. Wong, C.M., Atkinson, R.W., Anderson, H.R., Hedley, A.J., Ma, S., Chau, P.Y.-K., and Lam, T.H., A tale of two cities: effects of air pollution on hospital admissions in Hong Kong and London compared, *Environmental Health Perspectives*, 110(1), 67, 2002.

32. Environmental Protection Department, *API and Air Quality*, 2000. Available: www.info.gov.hk/epd/english/environmentinhk/air/air_quality/air_quality.html [Accessed on August 5, 2002].

33. Lloyd, O.L., Wong, S.L., Yu, T.S., and Wong, T.W., Mortality mapping in Hong Kong, 1979–83 and 1984–88: feasibility study and the patterns of cancers, Asia Pacific Journal of Public Health, 8(2), 66, 1995.

34. Bowling, A., *Research Methods in Health: Investigating Health and Health Services*, Open University Press, Philadelphia, PA, 1997.

35. Choi, K.H., *Geographical Analysis of Cancer Incidence and Mortality in Hong Kong Using Geographic Information System*, M.Phil. thesis, Chinese University of Hong Kong, 1998.
36. Jerrett, M., Eyles, J., and Cole, D., Socioeconomic and environmental covariates of premature mortality in Ontario, *Social Science and Medicine*, 47(1), 33, 1998.
37. Brewer, C.A., Basic mapping principles for visualizing cancer data using geographic information systems *(GIS), American Journal of Preventive Medicine*, 30(2, Suppl. 1), S25, 2006.

7

Initiating a GIS Project in Spatial Epidemiology

7.1 Introduction

Spatial patterns of diseases are often complex and intricate. We have seen from previous chapters and illustrations that spatial epidemiological methods can not only capture and identify gross and simplistic patterns but also can assist in the evaluation of disease risks and offer etiologic insights. Using geography to study disease or health care topics stems from the need to appreciate and recognize factors causing nonuniformity of disease distribution. These factors may include human (e.g., genetic, demographic, social, economic, cultural) and ecological (e.g., physical, environmental) bases of the disease setting. Because humans have difficulty examining and visualizing possible spatial associations in tabular displays, GIS performs a vital role in facilitating spatial understanding of multiple epidemiological factors to reveal trends, dependencies, and interrelationships that may not be observed as readily in the tabular formats.[1,2]

Person, place, and time are the three basic elements of epidemiology and outbreak investigations, and GIS allows the integration of all these elements onto a single platform. With the ever-growing demand of the public's right to know about environmental and community health matters, there is a pressing need to have more timely and effective response systems to address the present and changing conditions, as well as deliver early warnings on intervention and preventive measures. We are aware of the potential advantages of GIS over the conventional methods in health care analysis, surveillance, and planning. The potential applications of GIS in spatial epidemiology are limitless and await further exploration and research.

GIS development and applications should focus on cost-effective technologies tailored to user *needs*. Adaptation of learning experiences in using a GIS as spatial epidemiological approaches for medical care and disease analyses often involves two major steps: (1) setting up a GIS infrastructure and (2) conceptualizing a GIS project in the context of spatial epidemiology.

7.2   Setting Up a GIS Infrastructure

The GIS infrastructures needed to support applications in spatial epidemiology and health studies are discussed in Chapter 1. They include equipment (i.e., hardware and software), data, people, organization or institution, and methods or models (Table 7.1). However, details of these infrastructures require careful deliberation on resource implications and application needs. We list a few pertinent questions regarding the relevance of GIS applications (Figure 7.1):

i. How urgent are your needs and how often must you address them, that is, are these needs a one-time or repeated requirement?

If the needs are either urgent or for a one-time only event, then it is probably not the right time or opportunity to initiate a GIS project.

ii. For needs not of an urgent nature, can they be better handled by the introduction of GIS, that is, would existing personnel accept GIS being introduced and how much do these individuals know about GIS?

If existing personnel are not ready for GIS that should ultimately benefit the operation of your organization, then it may be necessary to hire outside help and buy some time for training and redevelopment of personnel.

iii. Do you need a GIS that provides simple drafting aids or supports highly sophisticated spatial analyses?

The former has simple and affordable solutions. The latter is often costly and demands a more elaborate approach and longer development time.

iv. Are data (preferably digital spatial) available for your GIS needs?

TABLE 7.1

GIS Infrastructures

Components	Explanation
Hardware	The computer on which a GIS operates
Software	Tools for the input and manipulation of geographic information, including DBMS
	Tools that support query, analysis, and visualization
	Graphic interface for users to access the system
Data	Geographic data and related tabular data
People/ institution	The thinking explorers who manage and develop GIS strategies for problem solving
Methods or models	GIS models and operational rules applicable to real-world exercises

One needs to start by investigating existing spatiotemporal data, including their geographic coverage, the available scales, data quality, and any barriers to access them (e.g., data protection as well as privacy and confidentiality issues). Failure to locate suitable data may become a significant obstacle to GIS adoption because embarking of GIS data development may be prohibitively costly and counterproductive if not planned properly.

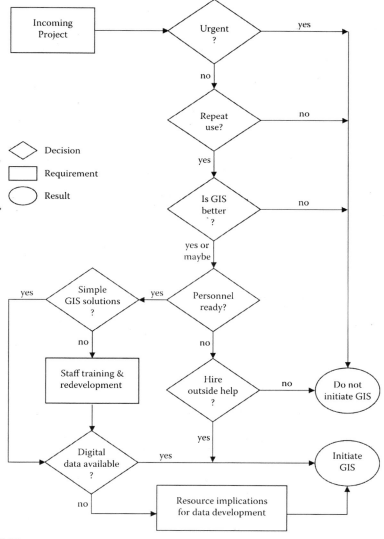

FIGURE 7.1
Considerations for a GIS project initiation.

Among the GIS infrastructures, hardware and software are comparatively the least problematic of all considerations. Usually, a GIS establishment for an expanded collection of functionalities will require a higher investment in both hardware and software. An organization will likely choose the affordable combination. Methods and models have become less of an issue because systems nowadays can support and facilitate interchange between an assortment of popular data structures and file formats. The deciding factors assuming organizational support, therefore, are the people and the data.

Never underestimate the internature and multinature as well as the interorganizational and intraorganizational cooperation of health informatics and GIS! Besides securing personnel skillful in GIS operation, a successful GIS program depends on a wide range of knowledge and expertise drawn from multiple contributing disciplines and on effective collaboration and teamwork. It is noteworthy that applications should guide and underscore the needs for any new data acquisition and personnel development. An overemphasis on data and metadata (data about data) development without practical and useful spatial applications around these data will not only impede further development but the data will also end up becoming useless and a waste of resources.

Because GIS adoption is for the long-term benefit of an organization, it is prudent to begin with a pilot configuration based on a project of a smaller scope. This approach offers an opportunity to test the waters at the outset and without jeopardizing the investment. Projects of a smaller scope will also facilitate the realization of project outcomes at an earlier stage and accelerate the completion of a project life cycle evidenced by cost–benefit analysis.

7.3   Conceptualizing a GIS Project

Tomlinson[3,4] and Briggs[5] offered a methodological approach to GIS systems design and implementation that resembles steps advocated in the data management field. The steps are essentially (1) needs assessment (strategic purpose, plan for the planning, determine technological requirements), (2) conceptual design (determine the end products, define the system scope), (3) physical design (create a data design, choose a data model, determine systems requirements), and (4) implementation (analyze benefits and costs, make an implementation plan).

The following discussion pertains to GIS developments in the areas of the geography of disease and health care systems, as described in the previous chapter. A two-tier procedure is recommended: (1) determining the focus of a GIS development and (2) conceptualizing a GIS application in epidemiology.

7.3.1   Determining the Focus of a GIS Development

In general, the focus of a GIS development will vary according to four aspects: setting, need, status quo, and operation.

  i. Setting: Who you are or for whom you are working

   A self-employed or private business setting (e.g., clinics, consultants) will have more freedom for choice, whereas a government or public department (e.g., Department of Health, Hospital Authority) may be bound by legislative mandates and interdepartmental policies.

  ii. Need: What is required

   The department involved should use data on hand to filter information or seek expert advice for decision makers to devise a plan of implementation (including cost, time frame, organizational structure, or restructuring, etc.).

  iii. Status quo: The types of equipment, data, and personnel you have on hand

   An updated list of inventories about equipment, data, and personnel will need to be compiled to estimate the extent of equipment upgrade, data acquisition, and personnel training or hiring.

  iv. Operation: The level of GIS operational skills

   Which types of spatial analysis are likely conducted in view of the applications: disease mapping, spatial overlay, geostatistical analysis?

The first three aspects are unique for each situation. The final aspect on GIS operation, however, should be considered with careful regard to the application settings. The types of spatial analysis should be commensurate with the operational skills of the technical staff. Three levels of analysis in increasing order of technical and operational competence are possible[6,7]: (1) *disease mapping* — a form of elementary analysis involving simple visual inspection of the chosen phenomenon, (2) *spatial overlay and related procedures* — more complicated operational skills including buffer and cluster analysis to identify possible hot spots[8], and (3) *geostatistical analysis* — requires contextual knowledge and sophisticated reasoning to explain relationships between geographic phenomena. All three levels of analysis may be called upon for a project but a logical progression from the simple to the more challenging tasks is recommended.

7.3.2   Conceptualizing a GIS Application

The procedure for the conceptualization of a GIS application in spatial epidemiology follows a five-stage process (Figure 7.2), which can be further

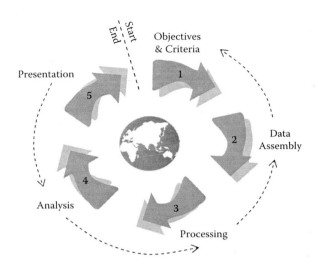

FIGURE 7.2
Conceptualizing a GIS application.

subdivided (Table 7.2). Although the five stages are logically sequenced (as indicated by the inner ring of numbered arrows in Figure 7.2), their execution requires some forward thinking (as indicated by the outer ring of arrows in the reverse direction). This is because advance knowledge of the expected outcomes of the GIS analysis is fundamental to determining the appropriate input data for these procedures. We must have a vision of the ultimate results to know the types of data to feed into the system to generate the desired outputs.

Table 7.2 summarizes the steps to contrive an idea and work out the procedures in achieving the goals. Note that the most elaborate of all stages occur at the beginning. Stages 1 and 2 have been expanded to include finer processing steps as described below.

Stage 1: Objectives and criteria involve laying down key epidemiological concerns of a GIS application.

The ability to structure an epidemiological question with a spatial context and a clear focus pretty much dictates the success of the GIS approach. A few brainstorming sessions to address the following points may be needed to identify objectives and criteria of the GIS development.

1. Ask and formulate a question in epidemiology.

   It is important to begin with a general statement or purpose of study. Very often, the purpose tends to be broad and involves the spatial distribution of a disease.

2. Examine whether it has a spatial context (so that GIS can be applied to it).

Clearly, all disease incidences can be mapped, but the concern here is to what degree? Determine, with reference to Chapter 2, the data type (point- or area-based) and the need for geocoding. Think about and visualize the types of map outputs (with reference to examples in Chapters 4–6) you would expect from the analysis.

3. Narrow down the focus.

What are the criteria or variables used in the study? Is there a factor of particular interest worthy of in-depth investigation?

4. Define the geographic extent and study period.

TABLE 7.2

Key Stages in the Conceptualization of a GIS Project

	Conceptualization	Explanation	Example(s)
Objectives and criteria	1. Ask and formulate a question in epidemiology	Identifying all key issues, concepts, and themes Organizing a narrative description of phenomenon	Spatial distribution of leukemia or cholera
	2. Examine whether it has a spatial context	Can the problem be visualized? What will be the method of symbolization?	Have residential locations or addresses of leukemia or cholera incidence
	3. Narrow down the focus	Constructing categories or themes across data Frame your questions and define your criteria Specify how and who will use the analysis	The relationship between childhood leukemia and nuclear power plants John Snow suspected in 1854 that cholera was a waterborne disease The problem should not be complicated with other issues
	4. Define the geographic extent and study period	Determine the geographic boundaries for the region of interest Select the appropriate map scale (resolution, precision, accuracy) Consider the duration of data for the investigation	Leukemia: Northern England and 1965–1985 for longer-term impact study Cholera: city of London in 1854 during the outbreak
	5. Develop hypotheses about the problem	Sort out connections between variables List specific hypothesis of spatial dependence Speculate predictions of large-scale trends or local effects	Were there higher risks of leukemia if patients lived near nuclear power plants over a length of time? Was there a higher incidence of cholera for residents obtaining water from a certain source?

—continued

TABLE 7.2 (Continued)

Key Stages in the Conceptualization of a GIS Project

	Conceptualization	Explanation	Example(s)
Data assembly	6. Assemble data from relevant sources	Acquire existing data about disease incidence and related variables Other supporting data (e.g., base map, census data) Be aware of MAUP	Find disease data from government sources and local practitioners Base map and census data from relevant government agencies or self-developed data
	7. Study data and assess their suitability	Immersion in the raw data (or a pragmatic selection of the data) Rearrange the data according to appropriate parts of the thematic framework Check for errors and omissions Understand metadata	Leukemia incidence and locations of nuclear power plants on a boundary map of Northern England Cholera incidence and locations of water pumps with streets of London as the reference base
	8. Include only data of direct relevance		
Processing	9. Determine GIS processes to be involved	Import/convert files Define coordinate systems and match projections Update spatial and attribute data Generate symbology and explore data	Point pattern if coordinates of events available Spatially continuous or surface analysis? Area if values of polygonal zones available
Analysis	10. Chart out sequences of analyses and queries	Consider the objectives and requirements of the analyses Select by location or attributes Perform buffers, overlay, modeling Consider the types of cartographic and analytical outputs	Occurrences by district or through time? Proximity or the situation nearby? Demographic analysis on who are most likely infected? Statistical or network analysis?
Presentation	11. Present results in maps and render your interpretation	Design maps and write reports The process of mapping and interpretation is influenced by the original research objectives as well as by the themes that have emerged from the data themselves	Leukemia: drew circles with sizes proportional to disease incidence Cholera: used points to represent respectively disease cases and water pumps and lines for roads

Delineate the area and period of study. These considerations have consequential effects on a suitable map scale and the representativeness or generalizability of the results.

5. Develop one or more hypotheses about the problem or issue you would like to test through your geographic inquiries and analyses.

Is it possible that the disease can be explained with particular environmental or socioeconomic factors? Visual displays of data using scatter plots or maps are a form of data exploration that often provide clues for generating hypotheses. Some GISs allow the exploration of spatial patterns in an interactive fashion.[6]

Stage 2: Data assembly is about finding suitable data to support the hypothesis testing established in Stage 1 above.

Two types of data are essential: (1) disease and related variables for hypothesis testing and (2) supporting data for visualization and presentation. These data are available either in the digital or nondigital (printed) format; otherwise, they must be collected or created by the project initiator. Locate as much as possible digital data that are ready for consumption to reduce the effort in creating your own data. The likely sources of digital data with credibility include government agencies and private developers.

6. Assemble data from relevant sources.

Digital data have become more accessible today, although their sources may be scattered. It makes sense to identify local clearinghouses and government agencies that carry and distribute digital spatial and nonspatial data to reduce duplication of efforts.[9] Although open access to databases of information generated by the research community can synergize individual efforts, data from unpublished sources must be carefully scrutinized for their reliability.

7. Study data and assess their suitability.

Not all data gathered may be suitable or required for the study. More often than not, quantitative data are less ambiguous in nature, whereas qualitative data must have the use of terminologies assessed against the application on hand. Check the metadata, if available, for information contents of positional and attribute data, reliability and quality assurance indicators, and dates of data. Where similar data are available from two or more agencies, select the one prepared by agencies of more credibility and better reputation.

8. Include only data of direct relevance.

The saying "garbage in garbage out" reflects this sentiment. Do not include data beyond what is required of the analysis.

As indicated in Section 2.3 of Chapter 2, the ideal data for spatial epidemiological research would comprise accurate and individualized accounts of the population of a study region, which are often untenable in many application environments. Such is the case for Hong Kong and most developing countries because of the different health care institutional settings. Data sources vary from country to country. Although the Department of Health keeps the disease and hospital admission data in the United Kingdom, both the Department of Health and the Hospital Authority of Hong Kong are entrusted with the duty of data collection. A lack of literature about the sources of available health data in Hong Kong makes the choice of health data difficult.

Figure 7.3 offers a guideline for determining data requirements for health studies in Hong Kong. The first step involves a decision on the measures of analyses or, more specifically, the mortality or morbidity aspects of a disease in relation to the population. Death is well documented in the many developed countries, and the number of deaths by each disease in Hong Kong has been recorded in statistical reports of the Hospital Authority since 1995. The statistics are also available in aggregated format by the Tertiary Planning

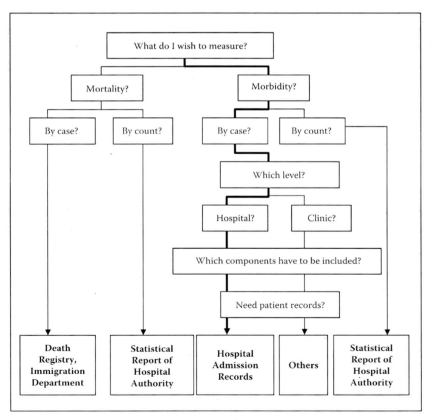

FIGURE 7.3
Guidelines for determining data requirements for health studies in Hong Kong.

Units (TPUs). Lloyd et al.,[10] for example, used these mortality data to produce the first atlas of disease for Hong Kong.

The second step requires a decision on whether individual (case) or aggregated (count) analysis is desired. Aggregated data do not contain case addresses of diseases, which are of paramount importance to enabling point pattern analyses or studies on disease spread. In general, mortality data are comparatively easier to obtain than morbidity data. It can be argued that if only the mortality data were examined, the truth would not be disclosed adequately.[11] Although health records from private clinics are available in Hong Kong, data inconsistency and privacy issues often preclude this option. Hospital admission records thus become the only health data available for health research in many instances.

*Stage 3: Processing encompasses working out all procedures
necessary to convert, align, and touch up data, including
simple visualization and data exploration techniques.*

9. Determine the GIS processes to be involved.

This step basically takes data gathered from Stage 2 and spells out the steps for data import and transfer. A number of GIS procedures may be necessary to align, clean up, and standardize data from different sources before they are operable under a unified setting. For example, vector layers and raster images must be georeferenced to superimpose on each other, new occurrences of infection must be added to the database, and recovered/deceased cases must be archived. The use of a map engine is also necessary to publish geographic data on the Web.

To facilitate data analysis in the next stage, it is essential to spend some time examining the data on hand. This step will involve simple visualization (i.e., displaying data using a variety of mapping techniques) and data exploration (i.e., using descriptive statistics and correlation analysis to inspect the data). A better understanding of the data, their properties, and relationships will assist the formulation of germane spatial queries, analytical objectives, and research hypotheses.

*Stage 4: Analysis involves charting out and executing
spatial queries and analytical sequences.*

Although proficiency in GIS operation is critical, it is important to remember that some GIS algorithms may be flawed. Therefore, intermediate results must be examined to correct for possible errors and prevent propagation of errors down the chain of command executions.

10. Chart out sequences of analyses and spatial queries.

Spatial analysis and query are attempted to address questions of what, where, when, why, and how (Table 7.3). The ability to convert problems or specific project criteria into GIS analysis steps relies on an individual who is capable of logical thinking and knows the tools and techniques on spatial data.

Start with setting up a problem statement and project criteria. At the elementary level, examine disease occurrences by geographic areas (e.g., districts, counties) and for different periods. At the contextual or associative level, examine the situation nearby (proximity analysis) and assess who are most likely affected (spatial autocorrelation of demographic and socioeconomic variables). At the modeling or prediction level, create risk surfaces (spatial interpolation) and estimate disease trends or movements (geostatistical modeling and network analysis).

Stage 5: Presentation includes report writing and map
presentation, as illustrated in Figure 3.5 of Chapter 3.

Because the end product of a spatial query or GIS analysis is often a map, the answer needs a context for its interpretation. For example, the question on "how extensive or how far was the spread of a disease" will require a display with disease spread showing area boundaries, roads, and prominent landmarks for place identification. Perhaps, a photograph of the area or the event timeline would add to the context. How much of these additional or peripheral data to add such that they are complementary instead of overpowering is not an exact science.

11. Present results in maps and render your interpretation.

The process of mapping and interpretation is often influenced by the original research objectives and by the themes emerging from the

TABLE 7.3

Examples of Spatial Queries and Analyses

Type	Spatial Examples	GIS Operations
What	What is there in location "A"?	Query of attribute data at location "A"
Where	Where can we find occurrences of "B"?	Select from an attribute all occurrences of "B" to map its spatial distribution
When	When did the pattern become significant?	Spatiotemporal mapping and spatial statistics
Why	Why was "C" found near "D" and was it affected by "E"?	Spatial overlay and autocorrelation plus substantive knowledge
How	How extensive or how far was the spread of "F"?	Spatial distribution and spatial measurements

data themselves. Proper assignment of graphic symbolization (color, text, legend, scale) can emphasize the visual impact of the query results and convey more effectively the intended message. Although software defaults may be a convenient means of delivering acceptable outputs, a good cartographic design can make a marked difference in guiding its readers to focus on the more important features and in making map reading more intuitive.

Once the appropriate analytical procedures, format of report writing, and map design have been worked out for an application to be repeated in cycle (e.g., a weekly surveillance account on a disease), the working sequence or templates should be programmed to standardize these processes. Over time, a collection of customized modules will be available to sustain the continuous implementation and facilitate procedural updates of a variety of application functions.

7.4   Signs of an Unfeasible Project

Not unlike other technology projects, GIS projects are costly to implement. It does not make good sense therefore to undertake a GIS project by trial and error with more than 80% of surveyed projects reportedly exceeding the budget.[12,13] This section contains some cautionary advice abstracted from major references[13-16] on unfeasible projects that should not be initiated because of a substantial potential for failure.

1. Major political issues are unresolved by the feasibility or pilot study.

    A GIS project is hardly an isolated case because it needs to make use of data and expertise from various sources. Interoperability of data and systems coupled with intraagency and interagency cooperation may present significant political challenges that may become obstacles to GIS initiatives.

2. Risks are too high.

    The majority of GIS infrastructures (i.e., equipment, data, people, organization or institution, and methods or models) are not in place nor do they have a clear focus. The probability of adverse consequences as a result of organizational, technical, or economic impediments is deemed too high.

3. The cost–benefit ratio is not favorable, particularly when benefits are intangible.

Costs for equipment, data, and staff are easily accountable, but the benefits of GIS in terms of productivity, efficiency, sustainability, and standardization are not directly measurable. These benefits are at best estimates and not very persuasive because they cannot be compared with other competing alternatives to identify the best use of resources.

4. Experience and training of existing staff are insufficient for the project.

Although it may be tempting to hire outside consultants to initiate a GIS project, the approach is a one-off solution and not sustainable. A longer-term alternative would rely on having capable in-house staff to continue with operating and enhancing the GIS applications.

5. Requirements or objectives are unclear and expected to change radically during the project phases.

Davis and Olson[17] affirmed that "strategies are general approaches for achieving an objective; methods are the detailed means for doing it." Although it is acceptable that people may not see reality in the same way, the objectives of a project certainly form the basis of a work strategy and selection of an appropriate methodology. Given the resource implication of a GIS project, it is prudent to have clear objectives at the outset because subsequent modifications may be prohibitively costly, as typified by the project diamond whose shape will be skewed given the changes made in any of its components.[13]

6. Lack of support from the senior management and executive levels.

Support from the management and executive levels is vital to GIS implementation. Issues of cost, training, and sharing of resources across agencies need management and executive decisions. It is not news that many GIS projects attributed their failures to a lack of organizational support.[16] It is ironic that the best way to gain support is to demonstrate successes, but there will not be any success story to tell if a GIS project cannot be initiated in the first place.

Rocheleau[16] also emphasized that the causes of many information system failures were due to poor project management, overwhelming complexity of systems, or technical problems. A checklist (Table 7.4) has been compiled in view of the above discussions to provide some guidance on the issues to be considered in the implementation of a GIS project.

TABLE 7.4

A Checklist for the Implementation of a GIS Project

Equipment		
Hardware		Hard drive capacity
		Backup and data exchange
		Processing capacity
		Video display requirement
		Peripheral devices (digitizer, scanner, printer, plotter)
		Stand-alone or network
Software		Desktop or workstation
		Single copy or floating
Data		
Standards		Coordinate referencing systems
		Accuracy requirements
		Naming conventions (data files, feature descriptions)
		Tiling or data subsets
		Metadata
Layers		Base map
		Other feature layers
Operation		Update and maintenance cycles
		Error tracking and correction
		Audit trails
People		
Administrator		Support for GIS work?
GIS operator		GIS competencies
		Project management skill
		How many?
Computer technician		Technical ability
		Programming ability
Organization/institution		
Commitment		Staffing
		Funding
Relationships		Interdepartment
		External groups
		Cooperative models
Service delivery		Establish priorities
		Control expectations
		Security and archiving
		Legal matters (copyright, liability, charging for access)
Methods/models		
Input		Primary data encoding method
		Sampling method
Process		Primary analytical procedures
Output		Primary map output
		Primary report types

7.5 Summary

Jacquez et al.[18] observed that the present-day spatial data analysis follows the 80-15-5 rule. That is, about 80% of effort is consumed in locating and inputting spatial data into the system; about 15% of the time is spent in data preprocessing, including format conversion and georectification; and only 5% of the undertaking is allotted to spatial analysis and modeling. Although we are making progress to revert this rule with better data sharing and easier-to-use systems with technological advances, it is not likely that an intelligent tool will be developed to tell us the "right" methods to use or the "right" buttons to press. The ultimate decision must come from the operators whose thinking process is guided by knowledge and experience founded on sound science and data.

It is important to note that no success is permanent and no failure is final. The most obvious approach to commence a GIS project is to get good and competent people for the job. "Find the right people and the job is half done" is certainly the motto to remember for GIS implementation. Hamil[13] identified six key competencies of a first-rate project manager worthy of consideration: (1) education and experience in project management, (2) negotiation and communication skills, (3) planning and organization skills, (4) effective problem solver, (5) leadership ability, and (6) aims for excellence in all work.

References

1. Rushton, G., Improving the geographical basis of health surveillance using GIS, in *GIS and Health*, Gatrell, A.G., and Loytonen, M., Eds., Taylor & Francis, London, 1998, Chap. 5.
2. Graham, A.J., Atkinson, P.M., and Danson, F.M., Spatial analysis for epidemiology, *Acta Tropica*, 91, 219, 2004.
3. Tomlinson, R., *Thinking About GIS: Geographic Information System Planning for Managers*, ESRI Press, Redlands, CA, 2003.
4. Tomlinson, R., *Planning for a GIS*, ESRI Press, Redlands, CA, 2001.
5. Briggs, R., *GIS Management & Implementation: The Challenges*, n.d. Available: http://www.utdallas.edu/~briggs/poec6383/introx.ppt [accessed on October 15, 2007].
6. Bailey, T.C., and Gatrell, A.C., *Interactive Spatial Data Analysis*, Longman Group, Essex, 1995.
7. Olson J., A coordinate approach to map communication improvement, *American Cartographer*, 3(2), 151, 1976.
8. Kingham, S., Gatrell, A.C., and Rowlingson, B., Testing for clusters of health events within a geographical information system framework, *Environment and Planning A*, 27, 809, 1995.

9. Rhind, D., Lessons learned from local, national and global spatial data infrastructures, in *Proceedings of National Geospatial Data Infrastructure (NGDI) Towards a Road Map for India*, Workshop, New Delhi, India, February 5–6, 2001. Available: http://www.gisdevelopment.net/policy/international/interna010pf. htm [accessed on October 15, 2007].

10. Lloyd, O.L., Wong, T.W., Wong, S.L., and Yu, T., *Atlas of Disease Mortalities in Hong Kong for the Three Five-Year Periods in 1979–93*, Chinese University Press, Hong Kong, 1996.

11. So, F.M., *An Application of Geographic Information Systems in the Study of Spatial Epidemiology of Respiratory Diseases in Hong Kong, 1996–2000*, M.Phil. thesis, Department of Geography, The University of Hong Kong, 2002.

12. Beynon-Davies, P., Human error and information systems failure: the case of the London ambulance service computer-aided despatch system project, *Interacting with Computers*, 11(6), 699, 1999.

13. Hamil, D.L., *Your Mission, Should You Choose to Accept It: Project Management Excellence*, 2001. Available: http://spatialnews.geocomm.com/features/mesa1/ hamil1.pdf [accessed on October 15, 2007].

14. Goodchild, M.F., and Kemp, K.K., Eds., *NCGIA Core Curriculum in GIS. Unit 67: Implementation Issues*, National Center for Geographic Information and Analysis, University of California, Santa Barbara, CA, 1990. Available: http://www. geog.ubc.ca/courses/klink/gis.notes/ncgia/u67.html [accessed on October 15, 2007].

15. Foote, K.E., and Crum, S.L., Project planning and life cycle, *The Geographer's Craft Project*, Department of Geography, The University of Colorado at Boulder, 2000. Available: http://www.colorado.edu/geography/gcraft/notes/lifecycle/ lifecycl_f.html [accessed on October 15, 2007].

16. Rocheleau, B., Governmental information system problems and failures: a preliminary review, n.d. Available: http://www.pamij.com/roche.html [accessed on October 15, 2007].

17. Davis, G.B., and Olson, M.H., *Management Information Systems, Conceptual Foundations, Structure, and Development*, 2nd ed., McGraw-Hill, New York, NY, 1985.

18. Jacquez, G.M., Greiling, D., and Kaufmann, A., *Spatial Pattern Recognition in the Environmental and Health Sciences: A Perspective*, GEOIDE Workshop, Quebec City, Canada, May 14–15, 2001. Available: http://www.spatial.cs.umn.edu/ CS8715/IM5_jacques_et_al.pdf [accessed on October 15, 2007].

8

Current GIS Research in Health Care and Disease Analyses

8.1 Geography of Health

The objective of spatial epidemiology is to identify the causes of diseases by correlating or relating spatial disease patterns to geographic variation in health risks, as we have demonstrated in previous chapters. We examine, in this chapter, the evolution, progress, and promising future developments in health care and disease analyses.

Health care studies are a hallmark of many academic disciplines. The concept of health is difficult to define. Historically, the term is used to denote the absence of diseases under a medical model that assumes scientific rationality using some objective and numerical measurements.[1-3] Under this model, however, illnesses based on subjective experience would not be accounted for. The functional model, meanwhile, contends that health and illness reflect the level of social normality rather than physical normality of individuals.[3,4] In the 1960s, the World Health Organization (WHO) defined health as "a state of complete physical, mental, and social well-being, not merely the absence of disease."[5] However, this idealistic and utopian definition has always been criticized and rejected for not being applicable in today's health care environment.[3,6,7]

The application of GIS methods in health and health care is a relatively new approach that started to gain acceptance in the 1990s.[7,8] We have seen from previous chapters a wide variety of methods for the mapping and analysis of disease data since the defining work of Cliff and Haggett.[9] Advances in new technologies have enabled the application of GIS in examining spatially related problems from many different perspectives. In addition to the descriptive mapping function, a GIS also is capable of data manipulation and geostatistical analysis.

The emphasis on spatial distribution and processes of various phenomena in geography contributes to the two research traditions in health geography: geography of disease and health care systems. The former concerns the description and understanding of the spatial variations in disease risks.[10] Health outcomes and epidemiological studies also include the more recent applications of GIS in near-real-time health and environmental surveillance or monitoring. The latter involves increasing applications of geographic analysis in health care delivery and planning.[11,12] These studies include the use of GIS methodology in the allocation or management of health services and resources.[13] There is also an increasing mix of the two traditions with applications involving the interface between epidemiological and health care delivery systems in relation to health care commissioning and needs assessment.

8.1.1   Health Outcomes and Epidemiological Studies

Because the visualization of map patterns can be the stimulus for generating hypotheses of disease causation,[14] epidemiologists have used maps to analyze associations among location, environment, and diseases. May[15] suggested this interaction as the relationship between pathological and geographic factors. Under this concept, the former (pathogen) refers to the causative agent, vector, intermediate, host, reservoir, and man, whereas the latter (geogen) encompasses the physical, human or social, and biological factors of the environmental context. How the geographic factors are correlated with the pathogens is the main focus in the ecology of disease. May,[16] Knight,[17] and Pyle[18] demonstrated that natural environmental explanations, particularly for vector-borne diseases, have been the strongest contribution in disease ecology.

The infamous John Snow study successfully applied the concept of spatial association in assessing health outcomes and disease prevalence.[5,19,20] Snow identified the outbreak of cholera by mapping the affected London water sources in 1854. The clustering of cholera near the wells supported Snow's hypothesis that cholera was a waterborne disease. Openshaw et al.[21] investigated cancer clusters and found common etiologic factors of scientific and media interest. In their study of the Sellafield region in England, they found the incidence of childhood leukemia to cluster near nuclear power plants.

With increasing urban population and industrialization, disease prevalence has changed and new diseases have emerged. By incorporating time and space with basic epidemiological concepts, the more recent applications involve near-real-time health and environmental surveillance or monitoring. Blanton et al.[22] reported a GIS-based and real-time Internet mapping for rabies surveillance to control the spread of wildlife rabies in the United States (restricted access for authorized users only at http://gis.cdc.gov/rabies/default.asp). To protect the health of Canadians, as well as to monitor and control the West Nile virus in Canada, the Public Health Agency of Canada has developed corresponding surveillance systems and infrastructure for West Nile virus surveillance[23] (see online system at http://www.cnphi-wnv.ca/healthnet/Mainpage.do). The fact that many recent occurrences of new and reemerging infectious diseases have originated in the Asia Pacific region also draws much interest to learning and knowing about disease surveillance and monitoring progress made in this region.[24] Such awareness is essential in promoting future global public health surveillance and coordination among the different international players.

8.1.2 Health Care Delivery Applications

Because research in the geography of health has focused on disease ecology and mapping studies, little attention has been paid to the study of health care resources and planning before the 1980s.[25] Research in the health care delivery system has been a new trend in the geography of health with two broad areas of study: (1) assessment of the accessibility and utilization of health care services and (2) evaluation of the spatial property of health care resources.[5,7,25,26]

The accessibility of health care resources has been examined largely by overlaying road network data and health care services in a GIS. Perry and Gesler[27] used the GPS in the development of a GIS to evaluate the accessibility of primary health care services in Andean Bolivia. They were convinced that GIS (through simple modeling in conjunction with field observations by GPS, along with satellite imagery and other pertinent health data) can help appraise and improve the physical accessibility of health care services in mountainous areas of developing countries. GIS was also applied to deal with emergencies. For instance, Kuiper et al.[28] monitored and planned emergency and ambulance services using a GIS. In addition, Mobley et al.[29] examined the relationships between market-level supply and demand factors of "ambulatory care sensitive conditions" among the elderly to determine if there was an impending shortage of physicians in the United States. They found that the existing supply of physicians was adequate, but their distribution across the landscape was less than optimal.

Policy planners for health care services have used GIS to select possible sites for building hospitals.[30,31] They also have evaluated the utility and accessibility of health care services by using the "location–allocation" model. Business managers use GIS to market their medical products.[20,32] Today, health services are managed more like conventional businesses that require the mapping and planning of service delivery within facilities. Economic and social factors are primarily used to analyze health care resource distribution in space and to study market penetration. Pharmaceutical marketers, for example, use spatial analysis and socioeconomic and demographic databases to identify areas of potential demand for their pharmaceutical products.[20] GIS has also been used to strategize the launching of new prescription drugs in the market and allocate spending in marketing activities.[33] The use of GIS and its spatial analysis functions has enhanced the marketers' ability to identify and characterize the stakeholders (patients, doctors, pharmacies, and medical facilities) to achieve a more accurate and detailed representation of need for services or for a particular product.[34]

In comparison, not much work has been done to determine and evaluate the effectiveness of intervention measures and international programs that have been introduced to combat diseases. With billions of dollars allocated to battling HIV/AIDS and avian influenza targeted at various countries worldwide, a study of the spatial coverage of the recipient communities and the achievements of the programs would help chart the path for future humanitarian efforts and possibly more effective allocation of resources. In a rare study, Tan[35] highlighted the use of GIS in monitoring and evaluating the HIV/AIDS programs in sub-Saharan African countries to assess needs measured in terms of disease prevalence compared with the amount of aid received by each country. It was found that countries receiving the largest amounts of aid were not the neediest and as much as 75% of the relief funds were for administrative expenses.

8.1.3   Health Care Commissioning and Needs Assessment

Health studies require different types of data because of the need to incorporate medical processes (patients, revenues, disease), facilities (hospitals, physicians, clinics), population (demographic, socioeconomic), cartographic features (administrative boundaries, referral areas, buildings, roads), environmental and natural resources (topographic, land uses, air, and water quality testing sites), remotely sensed landscapes (land cover, satellite images), and GPS-derived positions (self-collected coordinate data).[10,36] Tim[37] credited GIS for the integration of these data through the overlay operations. Curtis[38] demonstrated the use of GIS to store and manage data concerning population, health care, and finance. Here, geographic data, including the location of patients and hospitals, were used to overlay with the population census data for planning local health care services in East London.

GIS also is used as a tool in assisting medical clients deficient in a number of functional areas to achieve stability. The overlay approach in GIS is fundamental to providing health professionals timely and comprehensive information on complementary services available within a locality, for example, the siting of nutrition clinics to be located close to clinics for pediatric care.[39] Moreover, GIS supports the mapping of geographic proximity of patients and services to reduce travel time and cost and encourage collocation of health care provisions within a wider cross section of the community.[40,41] Collocation of health care provisions with other frequently used services (e.g., shopping, childcare, or work locations) not only yields benefits in terms of convenience in transport and travel but also reduces anxiety and stress levels of individuals caring for the patients.

Besides overlaying to examine the correlations of diseases and environment, GIS has also been used in simulating disease trend and spread based on different scenarios of population-based measures of access and behaviors. It is observed that GIS in epidemiology has two challenging needs.[42] The first is to reject the static view because meaningful inference about the causes of a disease is impossible without considering both the spatial and temporal aspects of disease manifestation. The second is to develop models to translate space–time data on health outcomes and related exposures into epidemiologically meaningful measures. The first need could be met by the design and implementation of space–time information systems for epidemiology,[43] while the second could be addressed by process-based disease models.

Predictive modeling of infectious disease spread using the GIS technology is an area that deserves more attention. It has been accepted in general that the transmission of many infectious diseases is influenced by climatic conditions. With increasing levels of concern over possible future impacts of climate change on human society, the development of climate-based disease early warning systems has been receiving more attention from the global community in recent years.[44] A study by Bell and Dallas[45] simulated the effects of fallout radiation from a nuclear explosion on U.S. populations and the health care systems of New York City, Chicago, Washington, DC, and Atlanta. They used multiple variables (including size of weapon, affected population, hospital data, weather and climate data) to estimate the impacts (including radiation dosage, casualties from fallout, combined injuries) under different scenarios. These simulations, despite limiting factors, nonetheless offered useful insights toward improving the accuracy of spatiotemporal models.

The simulation of an emergency event or a series of events to compare and contrast the results of epidemiological models can test the preparedness of emergency response systems. The preparedness exercise can help us plan better responses for casualty prioritization and treatment, considering limited medical resources available in the first few days after a catastrophic event. GIS used in tracking diseases and event simulation is essential in mobilizing emergency response resources to targeted areas in response to needs arising from outbreaks or disasters.[46] However, the use of geographic or spatial "intelligence" to manage health-related inventories and transactions is necessary in the events of threats or crisis. Better geographic analysis and IT infrastructure are indispensable in improving the flow and dissemination of critical information to decision makers who, in turn, can respond more swiftly and intelligently.

8.2 Contagious versus Noncontagious Disease Analyses

There is often confusion between the terms *infectious* and *contagious*. The following definitions are provided by the U.S. CDC[47]:

> *Infectious* disease — a disease caused by a microorganism and therefore potentially infinitely transferable to new individuals. May or may not be communicable. Example of *the noncommunicable variant* is a disease caused by toxins from food poisoning or infection caused by toxins in the environment, such as tetanus.

Communicable disease — an infectious disease that is contagious and can be transmitted from one source to another by infectious bacteria or viral organisms.

Contagious disease — a very communicable disease capable of spreading rapidly from one person to another by contact or close proximity.

In general terms, an *infectious* disease is spread through the air, whereas a *contagious* disease is spread by touch.[48] In medical terms, an infectious disease is one spread by germs (e.g., typhoid, typhus). Contagious refers to a disease spread by bodily contact (as with measles and human AIDS). A contagious disease (also called a communicable disease) is an infectious disease that is capable of being transmitted from a person or animal to another. In contrast, noncontagious diseases are those diseases that (usually) cannot be spread to another person (e.g., cancer, allergies, heart disease, diabetes).

Many methods for exploratory analysis of disease patterns are static and assume independence.[49] However, researchers have cautioned that these assumptions are often untenable because the real world is dynamic and things that are closer tend to be similar.[42] These methods are also not appropriate for infectious diseases because cases of infectious diseases are not independent (given that outcomes from subjects who live close to each other tend to be positively dependent) or static (because they move through time and space). Today, the unrealistic assumption of independence is substituted by tests for spatial autocorrelation,[50] and stationarity is dealt with by using spatiotemporal analysis and animation (Figure 8.1).[51,52] Attempts have been made to examine disease diffusion over time, in a large multistory residential complex (Figure 8.2).

Epidemiologists care about spatial effects of diseases and their developments because risk factors vary geographically. For noninfectious diseases, our attention tends to focus on identifying spatial association between diseases and certain risk factors. We often fail to measure all relevant risk factors because not all risk factors can be identified before a study is initiated. For infectious diseases, examination of spatial causation is critical given the potential for direct transmission between neighbors and near neighbors.

Our discussions above show that GIS is becoming a vital tool for scientists and public health officials in investigating the causes and spread of potentially deadly diseases, new or reemerging, around the world. The severe acute respiratory syndrome (SARS) outbreak in 2003 sent a worldwide signal that the threat of a global epidemic needed prompt actions to curb its spread. The global challenge of emerging infections has serious consequences for national and international laws because the spread of microbes is not contained by borders and boundaries. The globalization of infectious disease has made the use of GIS a necessity across the global health care system because outbreaks of infectious diseases such as SARS and avian influenza can be quickly analyzed by using GIS tools. International efforts are under way to better detect and respond to the threat of emerging infectious diseases. For

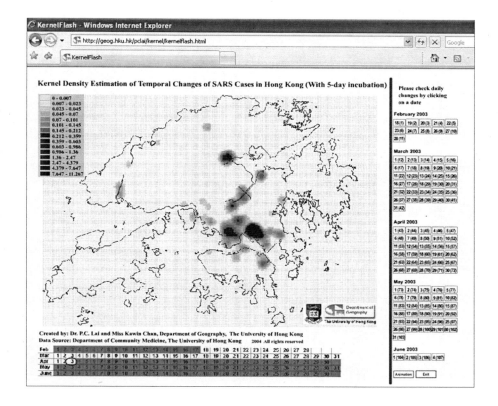

FIGURE 8.1
Spatiotemporal animation of the 2003 SARS outbreak in Hong Kong. Note: A screen shot of the
Web link at http://geog.hku.hk/pclai/kernel/ (log in with username "kernel" and password
"flash").

example, WHO and CDC have drafted action plans that stress and encourage the need to strengthen global surveillance of these diseases and allow
international communities to foresee, be aware of, control, and prevent their
spread.

8.3 Short-Term versus Long-Term
Surveillance and Disease Tracking

Disease surveillance is the process of monitoring diseases and involves the
continuous and routine collection of data related to health or exposures of
populations and the related analysis, interpretation, and dissemination of
the results. It is a century-long tradition in public health for the provision
of insights into disease causation and control. Global cooperation in disease

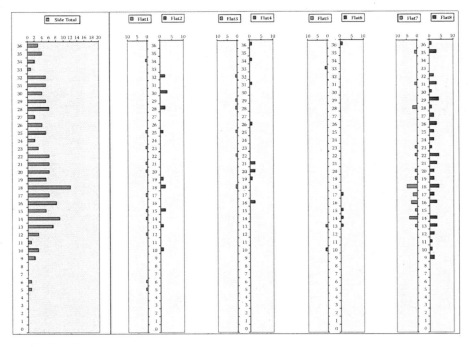

FIGURE 8.2
A cross-sectional analysis of the 2003 SARS outbreak in Hong Kong. Charts show SARS cases on April 15, 2003, based on a 5-day incubation period; the vertical charts show the floors or stories of Block E of the Amoy Garden with eight flats per floor; the leftmost chart shows cumulative cases on each floor from February 18 until April 15, 2003. The residents and the entire building were quarantined thereafter.

surveillance is increasingly valued by the international community particularly because a disease can emerge anywhere on the planet and spread quickly to other regions through trade and travel. The WHO declared in 1995 that emerging infections "represent a global threat that will require a coordinated and global response." One way of tackling the issue is through the WHO integrated disease surveillance program, which undertakes regular disease surveillance and offers real-time alert notification to its 192 member countries (as of 2007). Besides electronic sharing of laboratory and public health information databases, members are required to report immediately any emergence of diseases to ensure constant communication of suspected and confirmed outbreaks.

The purpose of disease surveillance is to improve the timeliness of information regarding threats to public health. International cooperation not only ensures electronic exchange of data on infectious diseases but also decreases the time to identify causes, risk factors, and suitable intervention measures to prevent a global outbreak. In terms of the transmission of infectious diseases, it is now evident that instead of relying on traditional assumptions that disease transmission occurs randomly in populations, contact patterns between susceptible and infected individuals, which are crucial to this process, have to be taken into account.[53] Dwolatzky et al.[54] found in their study that it was feasible to use a simple PDA/GPS device to locate the homes of patients who interrupted treatment and trace patients in areas without useful street maps. Studies on the theoretical and methodological framework of complex networks in recent years have also proven fruitful in understanding technological networks or networks of social interactions in disease surveillance.[55,56] In addition to the framework of complex networks, there has been a growing interest in designing spatial agent-based models where the contact patterns emerge from spatial simulations of the mobility of individuals.[57,58]

Geographic data are critical to environmentally influenced disease tracking for identifying hazards, monitoring distributions, and analyzing trends. The CDC announced in 2004 an initiative to link existing environmental and chronic disease data because the surveillance systems to date focus either on diseases/syndromes or on media (e.g., ambient air pollutants, toxic agents) without a formal linkage between them. Ritz et al.[59] reported that there is no existing blueprint for the longer-term surveillance of chronic illnesses in terms of coordination effort, enhancement of data collection methods, improved access to data, definition of standards, and better information dissemination to stakeholders. They provided arguments that effective surveillance does not always require formal linkage of exposure and health outcome data; indeed, there are problems inherent in surveillance of environmentally related diseases when based on formal linkage of routinely collected data.

Advances in GIS and related technologies have fostered new opportunities in examining diseases and their potential relations with environmental and other factors. Like many established statistical and quantitative methods, spatial epidemiological approaches are not free of bias. Even if the methods were flawless, which clearly is not the case, there remain some difficult challenges ahead before resolutions on global surveillance and international cooperation can be realized. These problems were echoed by Elliot and Wartenberg[10] to include concerns over data availability and quality, data protection, and confidentiality, and issues on exposure assessment, exposure mapping, and study design.

8.4 Summary

There is currently considerable interest in spatial epidemiology. From the perspective of public health, the spatial analysis of disease incidence can be of great benefit in reassuring citizens' concerns over local hazards and in monitoring the progress of prevention or intervention programs. The underpinning principle of public health is to promote the health of populations and not that of specific individuals. The primary strategy of public health is the prevention of disease and injury by changing the underlying conditions or the environment that place populations at risk through timely alerts of possible outbreaks and suitable intervention measures. GIS can offer an important means to explore areas that are vulnerable to disease and injury such that various alternatives of public health interventions may be assessed in the governmental context in which public health is practiced. There is naturally a parallel need to attend to the public's fear on matters concerning the confidentiality of health records and the protection of personal privacy.

There are, however, obvious deficiencies to the GIS approach. Graham et al.[60] raised some key issues needing immediate attention. The foremost concern is that spatial epidemiology creates numerous maps of risk that may be untestable or difficult to test satisfactorily. Measures of statistical uncertainty should be incorporated to provide appropriate validation tools for such spatial predictions. There is also the problem of choosing an appropriate spatial resolution and temporal dimension for a particular investigation. The current practice of presenting analytical results of different spatial resolution and temporal dimensions often confounds direct comparison of predictions made in competing studies.

Despite the criticism about the GIS approach as being retrospective, as opposed to being proactive to give early warnings as soon as an excess of disease occurrences is detected, the technique does hold distinct promise as a tool in the fight against emerging infectious diseases and other public health issues. Unfortunately, the application of a GIS requires careful planning, expense, training, and a steep learning curve, which can be an intimidating factor for its implementation. Cockings et al.[61] also warned that "the greatest need is for multidisciplinary research to use the most appropriate approach for each investigation, rather than that with which researchers are most familiar."

References

1. Jones, L.J., *The Social Context of Health and Health Work*, Macmillan, London, 1994.
2. Bowling, A., *Research Methods in Health: Investigating Health and Health Services*, Open University Press, Philadelphia, 1997.
3. Pol, L.G., and Thomas, R.K., *The Demography of Health and Health Care*, Kluwer Academic/Plenum Publishers, New York, NY, 2002.
4. Parsons, T., *The Social System*, Free Press, New York, NY, 1951.
5. Meade, M.S., Florin, J.W., and Gesler, W.M., *Medical Geography*, Guilford Press, New York, NY, 1988.
6. Gatrell, A.C., *Geographies of Health: An Introduction*, Blackwell, Oxford, 2002.
7. Meade, M.S., and Earickson, R.J., *Medical Geography*, Guilford Press, London, 2000.
8. Higgs, G., and Gould, M., Is there a role for GIS in the "new NHS"? *Health & Place*, 7, 247, 2001.

9. Cliff, A.D., and Haggett, P., *Atlas of Disease Distributions: Analytic Approaches to Epidemiological Data*, Blackwell, Oxford, 1988.

10. Elliot, P., and Wartenberg, D., Spatial epidemiology: current approaches and future challenges, *Environmental Health Perspectives*, 112(9), 998, 2004.

11. Kearns, R.A., Place and health: towards a reformed medical geography, *Professional Geographer*, 45(2), 139, 1993.

12. Kearns, R.A., Putting health and health care into place: an invitation accepted and declined, *Professional Geographer*, 46(1), 111, 1994.

13. Croner, C.M., Public health, GIS, and the Internet, *Annual Reviews of Public Health*, 24, 51, 2003. Available: http://www.cdc.gov/nchs/data/gis/GIS_AND_THE_INTERNET.pdf [accessed on October 15, 2007].

14. Lloyd, O.L., and Yu, T.S., Disease mapping: a valuable technique for environmental medicine, *Journal of Hong Kong Medical Association*, 46(1), 3, 1994.

15. May, J.M., Medical geography: its methods and objectives, *Geographical Review*, 40, 9, 1950.

16. May, J.M., *The Etiology of Human Disease*, M.D. Publications, New York, NY, 1958.

17. Knight, C.G., The geography of vectored diseases, in *The Geography of Health and Disease*, Hunter, J.M., Ed., University of North Carolina, Chapel Hill, NC, 1974, 46.

18. Pyle, G.F., *Applied Medical Geography*, Wiley, New York, NY, 1979.

19. Croner, C.M., Sperling J., and Bromme, F.R., Geographic Information System (GIS): new perspectives in understanding human health and environmental relationships, *Statistics in Medicine*, 5, 1961, 1996.

20. Lang, L., *GIS for Health Organizations*, ESRI Press, Redlands, CA, 2000.

21. Openshaw, S., Craft, A.W., Charlton, M., and Birch, J.M., Investigation of leukaemia clusters by use of a geographical analysis machine, *Lancet*, 1, 272, 1988.

22. Blanton, J.D., Manangan, A., Manangan, J., Hanlon, C.A., Slate, D., and Rupprecht, C.E., Development of a GIS-based, real-time Internet mapping tool for rabies surveillance, *International Journal of Health Geographics*, 5, 47, 2006.

23. Shuai, J.P., Buck, P., Sockett, P., Aramini, J., and Pollari, F., A GIS-driven integrated real-time surveillance pilot system for national West Nile virus dead bird surveillance in Canada, *International Journal of Health Geographics*, 5, 17, 2006.

24. Lai, P.C., and Mak, A.S.H., Eds., *GIS for Health and the Environment: Development in the Asia-Pacific Region*, *Lecture Notes in Geoinformation and Cartography*, Springer-Verlag, Berlin, 2007.

25. Howe, G.M., and Phillips, D.R., *Medical Geography in the United Kingdom, 1945–1982*, Academic Press, London, 1983.

26. McLafferty, S.L., GIS and health care, *Annual Reviews of Public Health*, 24, 25, 2003. Available doi:10.1146/annurev.publhealth.24.012902.141012 [accessed on October 15, 2007].

27. Perry, B., and Gesler, W., Physical access to primary health care in Andean Bolivia, *Social Science and Medicine*, 50, 1177, 2000.

28. Kuiper, J.A., Allison, T., Cilek, C.M., Miller, D.J., and Stache, J.E., Development of a GIS-based emergency planning system, in *Proceedings of Twentieth Annual ESRI User Conference*, San Diego, CA, 2000.

29. Mobley, L.R., Root, E., Anselin, L., Lozano-Gracia, N., and Koschinsky, J., Spatial analysis of elderly access to primary care services, *International Journal of Health Geographics*, 5, 19, 2006.

30. Dunn, E.D., Optimal routes in GIS and emergency planning applications, *Area*, 249(3), 259, 1992.
31. Peters, J., and Hall, B.G., Assessment of ambulance response performance using a geographic information system, *Social Science and Medicine*, 49, 1551, 1999.
32. Barnes, S., and Peck, A., Mapping the future of health future of health care: GIS applications in health care analysis, *Geographic Information Systems*, 4, 30, 1994.
33. Peled, R., Reuveni, H., Pliskin, J.S., Benenson, I., Hatna, E., and Tal, A., Defining localities of inadequate treatment for childhood asthma: a GIS approach, *International Journal of Health Geographics*, 5, 3, 2006.
34. Odoi, A., Wray, R., Emo, M., Birch, S., Hutchison, B., Eyles, J., and Abernathy, T., Inequalities in neighbourhood socioeconomic characteristics: potential evidence-base for neighbourhood health planning, *International Journal of Health Geographics*, 4, 20, 2005.
35. Tan, X., Evaluating HIV/AIDS Programs, *ArcUser Magazine*, ESRI Press, Redlands, CA, July–September 2006.
36. Waller, L.A., and Gotway, C.A., *Applied Spatial Statistics for Public Health Data*, Wiley, Hoboken, NJ, 2004.
37. Tim, U.S., The application of GIS in environmental health sciences: opportunities and limitation, *Environmental Research*, 71, 75, 1995.
38. Curtis, S., The development of GIS for locality planning in health care, *Area*, 21, 391, 1989.
39. Kendal, A., Peterson, A., Manning, M., Xu, F., Neville, L.J., and Hogue, C., Improving the health of infants on Medicaid by collocating special supplemental nutrition clinics with managed care provide sites, *American Journal of Public Health*, 92, 399, 2002.
40. Treadwell, H., and Ro, M., Community-based oral health prevention: issues and opportunities, *American Journal of Preventive Medicine*, 23(1, Suppl. 1), 8, 2002.
41. Sullivan, G., Kanouse, D., Young, A.S., Han, X., Perlman, J., and Koegel, P., Co-location of health care for adults with serious mental illness and HIV infection, *Community Mental Health Journal*, 42(4), 345, 2006.
42. Jacquez, G.M., Spatial analysis in epidemiology: nascent science or a failure of GIS? *Journal of Geographical Systems*, 2, 91, 2000.
43. Jacquez, G.M., Greiling, D.A., and Kaufmann, A.M., Design and implementation of a space-time intelligence system for disease surveillance, *Journal of Geographical Systems*, 7, 7, 2005.
44. WHO, *Using Climate to Predict Infectious Disease Outbreaks: A Review*, WHO/SDE/OEH/04.01, 2004. Available: http://www.who.int/globalchange/ publications/en/oeh0401.pdf [accessed on October 15, 2007].
45. Bell, W.C., and Dallas, C.E., Vulnerability of populations and the urban health care systems to nuclear weapon attack — examples from four American cities, *International Journal of Health Geographics*, 6, 5, 2007.
46. Pinto, A., Brown, V., Chan, K.W., Chavez, I.F., Chupraphawan, S., Grais, R.F., Lai, P.C., Mak, S.H., Rigby, J.E., and Singhasivanon, P., Estimating population size using spatial analysis methods, in *GIS for Health and the Environment: Development in the Asia Pacific Region, Lecture Notes in Geoinformation and Cartography*, Lai, P.C., and Mak, A.S.H., Eds., Springer-Verlag, Berlin, 2007, 271.
47. U.S. Centers for Disease Control and Prevention, *Controlling the Spread of Contagious Diseases: Quarantine and Isolation*, 2006. Available: http://www.redcross.org/preparedness/cdc_english/IsoQuar.asp [accessed on October 15, 2007].

48. McGraw-Hill, Infectious Disease, *Encyclopedia of Science and Technology,* McGraw-Hill, New York, NY, 2005.

49. Clarke, K.C., McLafferty, S.L., and Tempalski, B.J., On epidemiology and geo- graphic information systems: a review and discussion of future directions, *Emerging Infectious Diseases,* 2, 2, 1996. Available: http://www.cdc.gov/ncidod/ eid/vol2no2/clarke.htm [accessed on June 6, 2007].

50. Anselin, L., *An Introduction to Spatial Autocorrelation Analysis With GeoDa,* 2003. Available: www.sal.uiuc.edu/stuff/stuff-sum/pdf/spauto.pdf.

51. Lai, P.C., and Chan, K., *Kernel Density Estimation of Temporal Changes of SARS Cases in Hong Kong (With 5-Day Incubation), Spatio-Temporal Animation, 2004.* Available: http://geog.hku.hk/pclai/kernel/ (username: kernel; password: flash).

52. Lai, P.C., Wong, C.M., Hedley, A.J., Lo, S.V., Leung, P.Y., Kong, J., and Leung, G.M., Understanding the spatial clustering of severe acute respiratory syn- drome (SARS) in Hong Kong, *Environmental Health Perspectives,* 112(15), 1550, 2004.

53. Moonan, P.K., Bayona, M., Quitugua, T., Oppong, J., Dunbar, D., Jost, K.C., Jr., Burgess, G., Singh, K., and Weis, S., Using GIS technology to identify areas of tuberculosis transmission and incidence, *International Journal of Health Geo- graphics,* 3, 23, 2004.

54. Dwolatzky, B., Trengove, E., Struthers, H., McIntyre, J.A., and Martinson, N.A., Linking the global positioning system (GPS) to a personal digital assistant (PDA) to support tuberculosis control in South Africa: a pilot study, *Interna- tional Journal of Health Geographics,* 5, 34, 2006.

55. Boulos, M.N.K., Cai, Q., Padget, J.A., and Rushton, G., Using software agents to preserve individual health data confidentiality in micro-scale geographical analyses, *Journal of Biomedical Informatics,* 39(2), 160–170, 2006.

56. Colizza, V., Barrat, A., Barthelemy, M., and Vespignani, A., The role of the airline transportation network in the prediction and predictability of global epidem- ics, *Proceedings of the National Academy of Sciences of the United States of America,* 103(7), 2015, 2006.

57. Kho, A., Johnston, K., Wilson, J., and Wilson, S., Implementing an animated geo- graphic information system to investigate factors associated with nosocomial infections: a novel approach, *American Journal of Infection Control,* 34(9), 578, 2006.

58. Watkins, R.E., Eagleson, S.L., Beckett, S., Garner, G., Veenendaal, B., Wright, G., and Plant, A.J., Using GIS to create synthetic disease outbreaks, *BMC Medical Informatics and Decision Making,* 7, 4, 2007.

59. Ritz, B., Tager, I., and Balmes, J., Can lessons from public health disease surveil- lance be applied to environmental public health tracking? *Environmental Health Perspectives,* 113(3), 243, 2005.

60. Graham, A.J., Atkinson, P.M., and Danson, F.M., Spatial analysis for epidemiol- ogy, *Acta Tropica,* 91, 219, 2004.

61. Cockings, S., Dunn, C.E., Bhopal, R.S., and Walker, D.R., Users' perspectives on epidemiological, GIS and point pattern approaches to analysing environment and health data, *Health & Place,* 10(2), 169, 2004.

Appendix A

List of GIS Software

The following list is provided for reference only and is not meant to be exhaustive.

GIS/Image Processing Software	Source/Company	Remarks[a]
ArcGIS products ArcView	ESRI	www.esri.com; free ArcExplorer and ArcReader
AutoCAD Map 3D AutoCAD Mapguide	Autodesk	www.autodesk.com; free Autodesk Express Viewer and Volo View Express 2.01
CrimeStat	Ned Levine & Associates	www.icpsr.umich.edu/CRIMESTAT; distributed freely for educational or research purposes; GIS for the analysis of crime incident locations
ERDAS Imagine	Leica Geosystems	gi.leica-geosystems.com; free ERDAS ViewFinder 2.1
ER Mapper	ER Mapper	www.ermapper.com; free ER Viewer
GeoDa	Spatial Analysis Laboratory, University of Illinois	www.geoda.uiuc.edu; free program
Geomedia	Intergraph	www.intergraph.com; free Geomedia viewer
Geomatica	PCI Geomatics	www.pcigeomatics.com; free Geomatica FreeView
GRASS GIS	GRASS Development Team	www.geog.uni-hannover.de; free software released under GNU General Public License; originally developed by the U.S. Army Construction Engineering Research Laboratories
HealthMapper	WHO	www.who.int/health_mapping/tools/; GIS for disease surveillance and mapping applications; free upon request and special conditions
IDRISI	Clark Labs	www.clarklabs.org
MapInfo Professional	MapInfo	www.mapinfo.com; MapInfo ProViewer
Maptitude, TransCAD	Caliper	www.caliper.com; GIS for transport applications
TatukGIS	TatukGIS	www.tatukgis.com; free GIS viewer

[a] The links to GIS Web resources change periodically; more updated links are accessible from the GeoCommunity homepage at www.geocomm.com.

Appendix B
Data Description

Unless otherwise specified, the sample data sets used in this book were compiled and edited by the GIS research team of the Department of Geography of the University of Hong Kong. These data are solely for demonstration purposes and should not be taken as a reflection of the real situation. Users may acquire the official digital data from the respective agencies.

Hong Kong Special Administrative Region (HKSAR)	
Type of Data	**Sources**
Census data	Census and Statistics Department, HKSAR
Disease surveillance	Department of Health, HKSAR
Environmental	Environmental Protection Department, HKSAR
Hospital admissions	Hong Kong Hospital Authority
Maps of Hong Kong	Survey and Mapping Office, Lands Department, HKSAR
Thailand	
Type of Data	**Sources**
Disease surveillance	Bureau of Epidemiology of Thailand
Maps of Thailand	Royal Thai Survey Department via Bureau of Epidemiology of Thailand

TABLE B.1

Data Items of Asthma Cases in Hong Kong, 1996–2000

	Item	Type of Data	Mandatory (Y/N)	Description
1	REFNO	Text/numeric	Y	Case identifier (e.g., a unique record number)
2	SEX	Text	N	Sex of a patient
3	DOB	Date (dd/mm/ yyyy)	N	Date of birth of a patient
4	BLDG	Text/numeric	N	Building name of place of residence of a patient
5	X	Numeric	Y	Geocoded location of place of
6	Y			residence, using HK1980 grid coordinate system[a]
7	HOSP	Text	Y	Code of the hospital that admits the patient
8	ICD	Text	Y	International Classification of Disease in numeric codes (e.g., asthma, 493; bronchitis, 466, 490–491; pneumonia, 481–483, 485–486)
9	DOA	Date (dd/mm/ yyyy)	Y	Admission date of episode
10	DOD	Date (dd/mm/ yyyy)	Y	Discharge date of episode

Data source: Hong Kong Hospital Authority.

[a]*Refer to Section 2.1 of Chapter 2 for a brief description of the HK1980 grid coordinate system.*

TABLE B.2

Data Items of SARS Cases in Hong Kong, April 1 to May 15, 2003

	Item	Type of Data	Mandatory (Y/N)	Description
1	REFNO	Text/numeric	Y	Arbitrarily assigned and unique case number
2	B_NAME	Text/numeric	N	Building name of place of residence
3	BLOCK	Text/numeric	N	Block number of place of residence
4	STREET	Text/numeric	N	Street number of place of residence
5	X	Numeric	Y	Geocoded location of place of
6	Y			residence, using HK1980 grid coordinate system[a]
7	CDATE	Date (dd/mm/ yyyy)	Y	Date of confirmed SARS episode
8	CCOUNTS	Numeric	Y	Cumulative disease counts at the building level[b]

Data source: Various newspapers.

[a]*Refer to Section 2.1 of Chapter 2 for a brief description of the HK1980 grid coordinate system.*

[b]*The locations of patients were represented at the building level, and we counted the number of patients at this level of spatial detail.*

TABLE B.3

Data Items of Dengue Cases in Thailand, 2004

	Itemem	Type of Datata	Mandatory (Y/N)N)	Descriptionon
1	REFNO	Text/numeric	Y	Case identifier (e.g., a unique record number)r)
2	SEX	Text	Y	Sex of a patientnt
3	AGE	Numeric	Y	Age of a patientnt
4	RACE	Numeric	N	Race of a patient
5	OCCU	Numeric	N	Occupation of a patient
6	VILLAGE	Numeric	Y	Village code of a patient
7	TUMBON	Numeric	Y	Subdistrict code of a patient
8	AMPHOE	Numeric	Y	District code of a patient
9	CHANGWAT	Numeric	Y	Province code of a patient
10	HOSP	Numeric	Y	Hospital attending the patient
11	DS	Date (dd/mm/ yyyy)	Y	Date a patient fell sick
12	DD	Date (dd/mm/ yyyy)	Y	Date a patient was confirmed to have dengue
13	RES	Numeric	Y	Outcome of a patient (e.g., discharged from hospital; died; transferred)

Data source: Bureau of Epidemiology of Thailand.

TABLE B.4

Air Pollution Indices of Hong Kong, January 1999 to December 2000

	Items	Type of Data	Mandatory (Y/N)	Description
1	Feature type	Point	Y	The feature type of this file is point
2	Ref. no.	Text/numeric	Y	A unique identifier of individual pollution monitoring site
3	Pollution monitor address	Text	Y	Address of a pollution monitoring site
4	X	Numeric	Y	Geocoded location of a pollution monitoring site, using HK1980 grid coordinate system[a]
5	Y			
6	Average API	Numeric	Y	Mean of API values measured between 1999 and 2000
7	API 01/1999	Numeric	Y	Mean of API values for each day in 01/1999
8	API 02/1999	Numeric	Y	Mean of API values for each day in 02/1999
9	API 03/1999	Numeric	Y	Mean of API values for each day in 03/1999
10	API 04/1999	Numeric	Y	Mean of API values for each day in 04/1999
11	API 05/1999	Numeric	Y	Mean of API values for each day in 05/1999
12	API 06/1999	Numeric	Y	Mean of API values for each day in 06/1999
13	API 07/1999	Numeric	Y	Mean of API values for each day in 07/1999
14	API 08/1999	Numeric	Y	Mean of API values for each day in 08/1999
15	API 09/1999	Numeric	Y	Mean of API values for each day in 09/1999
16	API 10/1999	Numeric	Y	Mean of API values for each day in 10/1999
17	API 11/1999	Numeric	Y	Mean of API values for each day in 11/1999
18	API 12/1999	Numeric	Y	Mean of API values for each day in 12/1999
20	API 01/2000	Numeric	Y	Mean of API values for each day in 01/2000
21	API 02/2000	Numeric	Y	Mean of API values for each day in 02/2000
22	API 03/2000	Numeric	Y	Mean of API values for each day in 03/2000
23	API 04/2000	Numeric	Y	Mean of API values for each day in 04/2000

24	API 05/2000	Numeric	Y	Mean of API values for each day in 05/2000
25	API 06/2000	Numeric	Y	Mean of API values for each day in 06/2000
26	API 07/2000	Numeric	Y	Mean of API values for each day in 07/2000
27	API 08/2000	Numeric	Y	Mean of API values for each day in 08/2000
28	API 09/2000	Numeric	Y	Mean of API values for each day in 09/2000
29	API 10/2000	Numeric	Y	Mean of API values for each day in 10/2000
30	API 11/2000	Numeric	Y	Mean of API values for each day in 11/2000
31	API 12/2000	Numeric	Y	Mean of API values for each day in 12/2000

Data source: Environmental Protection Department, HKSAR.

[a]*Refer to Section 2.1 of Chapter 2 for a brief description of the HK1980 grid coordinate system.*

TABLE B.5

Tertiary Planning Units of Hong Kong, 1996

	Items	Type of Data	Mandatory (Y/N)	Description
1	Feature type	Point	Y	The feature type of this file is polygon
2	Ref. no.	Text/numeric	Y	A unique identifier of individual TPU
3	TPU code	Text	Y	A unique three-digit code assigned to each TPU (e.g., 111, 133) It can be used to aggregate data or link with other census data
4	Other variables	Text/numeric	N	Demographic and socioeconomic variables (e.g., age, occupation, income)

Data source: Census and Statistics Department, HKSAR.

TABLE B.6

District Councils of Hong Kong, 1996

	Items	Type of Data	Mandatory (Y/N)	Description
1	Feature type	Point	Y	The feature type of this file is polygon
2	Ref. no.	Text/numeric	Y	A unique identifier of individual DC
3	District Code	Text	Y	A unique 3-digit code assigned to each DC (e.g., 111, 133) It can be used to aggregate data or link with other census data
4	District Name	Text	N	Name of DC (e.g., Central and Western, Yau Tsim Mong, Wan Chai, Tuen Mun)

Data source: Census and Statistics Department, HKSAR.

TABLE B.7

Amphoe (District) Boundary

	Items	Type of Data	Mandatory (Y/N)	Description
1	Feature type	Point	Y	The feature type of this file is polygon
2	Ref. no.	Text/numeric	Y	A unique identifier of individual amphoe
3	Amphoe_code	Text	Y	Code of an amphoe (e.g., 1110)
4	Amphoe_name	Text	Y	Name of an amphoe
5	X_centroid	Text	Y	Longitude of the centroid of individual amphoe
6	Y_centroid	Text	Y	Latitude of the centroid of individual amphoe

Data source: Royal Thai Survey Department.

TABLE B.8

Changwat (Province) Boundary

	Items	Type of Data	Mandatory (Y/N)	Description
1	Feature type	Point	Y	The feature type of this file is polygon
2	Ref. no.	Text/numeric	Y	A unique identifier of individual changwat
3	Changwat_code	Text	Y	Code of a changwat (e.g., 45)
4	Changwat_name	Text	Y	Name of a changwat
5	X_centroid	Text	Y	Longitude of the centroid of individual changwat
6	Y_centroid	Text	Y	Latitude of the centroid of individual changwat

Data source: Royal Thai Survey Department.

Appendix C

Data Preparation in Microsoft Excel

The "pivot table" is a very useful function for processing and summarizing spatial data in Microsoft Excel. A pivot table can be used to sort, count, and summarize data stored in a spreadsheet and create a second table to store and display the summarized data. Users can set up and change the structure of the summary table by graphically dragging and dropping fields. The operation to summarize data by attribute is outlined below.

1. Open in Excel a database file containing disease records. [Note: Look for the DBF format if your disease data come as a shapefile.]
2. Find "Pivot Table" from the "Data" menu on the toolbar.
3. Choose "Microsoft Excel list or database" for the first question and choose "Pivot Table" for the second question.

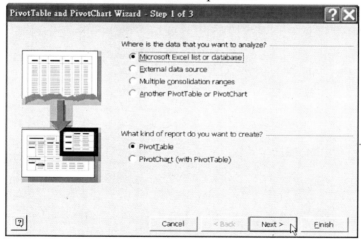

4. Highlight the attributes in your database to specify the source data of the pivot table.

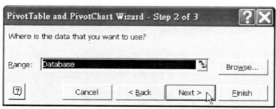

5. Choose "Layout" to design the data summary.

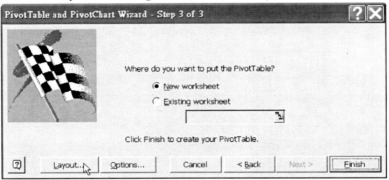

6. In the layout design window, move the attribute variable to base the summary on (e.g., DISTRICT name) to the column on the left and then move the variable that stores the unique reference number of your incident data (e.g., identification number of disease cases) to the column on the right, as illustrated in the figure below. You can change the calculation method of the variable by clicking once on the variable on the right column. Click OK when finished and a summary table will appear. The summary table can be imported into a GIS to carry out spatial analysis.

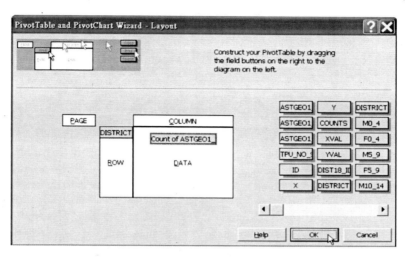

	A	B
1	Count of ASTGEO1	
2	DISTRICT ▼	Total
3	CENTRAL & WESTERN	562
4	EASTERN	626
5	ISLANDS	190
6	KOWLOON CITY	629
7	KWAI TSING	335
8	KWUN TONG	387
9	NORTH	408
10	SAI KUNG	256
11	SHA TIN	455
12	SHAM SHUI PO	707
13	SOUTHERN	265
14	TAI PO	426
15	TSUEN WAN	338
16	TUEN MUN	338
17	WAN CHAI	371
18	WONG TAI SIN	338
19	YAU TSIM MONG	773
20	YUEN LONG	724
21	Grand Total	8128

Note: The "count" method is suitable when each record represents a case in the attribute table. In instances where each record contains multiple occurrences (e.g., a record represents a building that may have more than one diseased individuals, as illustrated in the diagram below), the "sum" function of the pivot table should be used to add up the total. That is to say that the variable for the column on the right should be replaced by "sum" for the calculation. Another table will appear with a list of the sum of values (i.e., the total number of disease occurrences) by districts.

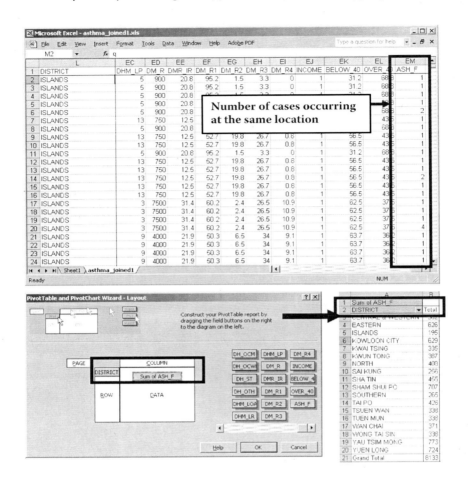

Appendix D

Useful Web References

Overviews and Guides to GIS

The Geographer's Craft, Department of Geography, University of Colorado at Boulder. Available: www.colorado.edu/geography/gcraft/contents.html.

Getting to Know Desktop GIS, Chapters 1–6. Available: http://www.geo.ntnu.edu.tw/faculty/hchou/class/gis/deskgis/ch1.htm,~/ch2.htm, ~/ch3.htm, ~/ch4.htm, ~/ch5.htm, ~/ch6.htm.

GIS Self-Learning Tool, Department of Geomatics, University of Melbourne. Available: http://www.geom.unimelb.edu.au/gisweb/.

GIS Tutorials, GIS Development. Available: http://www.gisdevelopment.net/tutorials/index.htm.

Modern Geographic Information System (CSS 411), Cornell University. Available: http://www.css.cornell.edu/courses/411/css411.html.

USGS and Science Education, USGS. Available: http://education.usgs.gov/.

Web-Based Tools for Public Health and Data Analysis

Health Map — Global Disease Alert Map, Children's Hospital Informatics Program, Harvard-MIT Division of Health Sciences & Technology. Available: http://www.healthmap.org/en.

Improving Public Health through Geographical Information Systems: an Instructional Guide to Major Concepts and Their Implementation, The University of Iowa. Available: http://www.uiowa.edu/~geog/health/.

Online Analytical Statistical Information System (OASIS), Georgia Department of Human Resources, Division of Public Health, Office of Health Information and Policy. Available: http://oasis.state.ga.us/ [accessed November 2007].

Web site for GIS Health Data, Stanford University, Available: http://www-sul.stanford.edu/depts/gis/medical.html.

Index